WITHOUT CONSCIENCE

WITHOUT

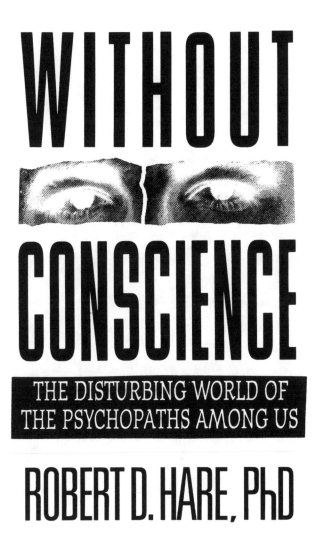

CONSCIENCE

THE DISTURBING WORLD OF THE PSYCHOPATHS AMONG US

ROBERT D. HARE, PhD

THE GUILFORD PRESS
New York   London

© 1993 by Robert D. Hare, PhD
Published in 1999 by The Guilford Press
A Division of Guilford Publications, Inc.
72 Spring Street, New York, NY 10012
http://www.guilford.com

Printed in the United States of America

This book is printed on acid-free paper.

Last digit is print number: 9   8   7   6   5   4   3

Library of Congress Cataloging-in-Publication Data

Hare, Robert D., 1934–
    Without conscience: the disturbing world of the psychopaths
among us / Robert D. Hare.
        p.   cm.
    Originally published: New York: Pocket Books, 1995.
    ISBN 1-57230-451-0 (pbk.)
    1. Antisocial personality disorders.   2. Psychopaths.   I. Title.
[RC555.H365   1998]
616.85'82—dc21   98-51786
                                                                CIP

Permission for letters appearing on pp. 192–193 granted by Ann
Landers and Creators' Syndicate

To the memory of my parents, Yvonne and Henry, and my sister, Charmaine

Contents

CONTENTS

Author's Note

Psychopathy is a personality disorder defined by a distinctive cluster of behaviors and inferred personality traits, most of which society views as pejorative. It is therefore no light matter to diagnose an individual as a psychopath. Like any psychiatric disorder, diagnosis is based on the accumulation of evidence that an individual satisfies at least the minimal criteria for the disorder. In cases based on my own files the individuals have been carefully diagnosed on the basis of extensive interview and file information. However, I have disguised these individuals by altering details and removing identifying information, without compromising the point I was trying to make.

Although the topic of this book is psychopathy, *not everyone described herein is a psychopath*. Many of the examples I use are taken from published reports, the news media, and personal communications, and I cannot be sure that the individuals in question are psychopaths, even though they may have been given the label by others. In each case, however, the documented evidence concerning some aspect of the person's behavior is either consistent with the concept of psychopathy or illustrates a key trait or behavior that is typical of the disorder. These individuals may or may not be psychopaths. But their reported behavior provides a useful vehicle for elaborating the various traits and behaviors that define psychopathy. *The reader should not assume that an individual is a psychopath simply because of the context in which he or she is portrayed in this book.*

Preface and Acknowledgments

Psychopaths are social predators who charm, manipulate, and ruthlessly plow their way through life, leaving a broad trail of broken hearts, shattered expectations, and empty wallets. Completely lacking in conscience and in feelings for others, they selfishly take what they want and do as they please, violating social norms and expectations without the slightest sense of guilt or regret. Their bewildered victims desperately ask, "Who are these people?" "What makes them the way they are?" "How can we protect ourselves?" Although these and related questions have been the focus of clinical speculation and empirical research for over one hundred years—and of my own work for a quarter-century—it is primarily within the last few decades that the deadly mystery of the psychopath has begun to reveal itself.

When I agreed to write this book I knew it would be difficult to present hard scientific data and circumspection in a way that the public could understand. I would have been quite comfortable remaining in my academic ivory tower, having esoteric discussions with other researchers and writing technical books and articles. However, in recent years there has been a dramatic upsurge in the public's exposure to the machinations and depredations of psychopaths. The news media are filled with dramatic accounts of violent crime, financial scandals, and violations of the public trust. Countless movies and books tell the stories of serial killers, con artists, and members of organized crime. Although many of these accounts and portrayals are of psychopaths, many others are not, and this important distinction is often lost on the news media, the entertainment industry, and the public. Even those members of the criminal justice system—lawyers, forensic psychiatrists and psychologists, social workers, parole officers, law enforcement officers, correctional staff—whose work daily brings them into contact with psychopaths often have little practical appreciation of the sort of people they are dealing with. This failure to distinguish between offenders who are psychopaths and those who are not has dire consequences for society, as this book makes clear. On a more personal level, it is very likely that at some time in your life you will come into painful contact with a psychopath. For your own physical, psychological, and financial well-being it is crucial that you know how to identify the psychopath, how to protect yourself, and how to minimize the harm done to you.

Much of the scientific literature on psychopathy is technical, abstract, and difficult to follow for those who lack a background in the behavioral sciences. My goal was to translate this literature so that it became accessible, not only to the general public but to members of the criminal justice system and the mental health community. I tried not to oversimplify theoretical issues and research findings or to overstate what we know. I hope that those readers whose interest is piqued will use the chapter notes to delve deeper into the topic.

The scientific slant to this book reflects my background in experimental psychology and cognitive psychophysiology. Some readers may be disappointed to see that I have devoted little space to discussions of psychodynamic issues, such as unconscious processes and conflicts, defense mechanisms, and so forth. Although many books and hundreds of articles on the psychodynamics of psychopathy have been written over the past fifty years, in my opinion they have not greatly advanced our understanding of the disorder. To a large extent, this is because most psychodynamic accounts of psychopathy have an armchair, often circular, quality about them and therefore do not readily lend themselves to empirical study. However, recently there have been some attempts to establish congruence between psychodynamic speculations about psychopathy and the theories and procedures of behavioral science. Some of the results of this work are interesting and, where relevant, are discussed in this book.

Over the years I have been blessed with a steady stream of outstanding graduate students and assistants. Our relationships have always been mutually beneficial: I provide guidance and a nurturing environment and they provide the fresh ideas, creative spark, and enthusiasm for research needed to keep a laboratory vibrant and productive. Their contributions are evident in the frequency with which graduate students are listed as senior authors on publications emanating from my laboratory. I am particularly indebted to Stephen Hart, Adelle Forth, Timothy Harpur, Sherrie Williamson, and Brenda Gillstrom, each of whom played a major role in my thinking and research over the past decade.

Our research has been supported by grants from the Medical Research Council of Canada, The MacArthur Research Network on Mental Health and the Law, and the British Columbia Health Research Foundation. Most of this research was conducted in institutions run by the Correctional Service of Canada. The cooperation of the inmates and staff of these institutions is gratefully acknowledged. To protect the identities of the inmates who took part in the research I have altered the details of specific cases or combined several cases into composites.

I would like to thank Judith Regan for encouraging me to write this book, and Suzanne Lipsett for showing me how to convert technical material into readable prose.

My view of life has been greatly influenced by the courage, determination, and grace of my daughter, Cheryl, and my sister, Noelle. I owe a special debt to my wife and best friend, Averil, who, in spite of a demanding professional career of her own, somehow found the time and energy to actively support and encourage my work. Her warmth, judgment, and clinical acumen have kept me happy, secure, and sane over the years.

WITHOUT CONSCIENCE

[G]ood people are rarely suspicious: they cannot imagine others doing the things they themselves are incapable of doing; usually they accept the undramatic solution as the correct one, and let matters rest there. Then too, the normal are inclined to visualize the [psychopath] as one who's as monstrous in appearance as he is in mind, which is about as far from the truth as one could well get.... These monsters of real life usually looked and behaved in a more normal manner than their actually normal brothers and sisters; they presented a more convincing picture of virtue than virtue presented of itself—just as the wax rosebud or the plastic peach seemed more perfect to the eye, more what the mind thought a rosebud or a peach should be, than the imperfect original from which it had been modelled.

—William March, *The Bad Seed*

Introduction: The Problem

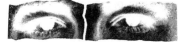

Several years ago two graduate students and I submitted a paper to a scientific journal. The paper described an experiment in which we had used a biomedical recorder to monitor electrical activity in the brains of several groups of adult men while they performed a language task. This activity was traced on chart paper as a series of waves, referred to as an electroencephalogram (EEG). The editor returned our paper with his apologies. His reason, he told us: "Frankly, we found some of the brain wave patterns depicted in the paper very odd. Those EEGs couldn't have come from real people."

Some of the brain wave recordings were indeed odd, but we hadn't gathered them from aliens and we certainly hadn't made them up. We had obtained them from a class of individuals found in every race, culture, society, and walk of life. Everybody has met these people, been deceived and manipulated by them, and forced to live with or repair the damage they have wrought. These often charming—but always deadly—individuals have a clinical name: *psychopaths*. Their hallmark is a stunning lack of conscience; their game is self-gratification at the other person's expense. Many spend time in prison, but many do not. All take far more than they give.

1

This book confronts psychopathy head-on and presents the disturbing topic for what it is—a dark mystery with staggering implications for society; a mystery that finally is beginning to reveal itself after centuries of speculation and decades of empirical psychological research.

To give you some idea of the enormity of the problem that faces us, consider that there are at least 2 million psychopaths in North America; the citizens of New York City have as many as 100,000 psychopaths among them. And these are conservative estimates. Far from being an esoteric, isolated problem that affects only a few people, psychopathy touches virtually every one of us.

Consider also that the prevalence of psychopathy in our society is about the same as that of schizophrenia, a devastating mental disorder that brings heart-wrenching distress to patient and family alike. However, the scope of the personal pain and distress associated with schizophrenia is small compared to the extensive personal, social, and economic carnage wrought by psychopaths. They cast a wide net, and nearly everyone is caught in it one way or another.

The most obvious expressions of psychopathy—but by no means the only ones—involve flagrant criminal violation of society's rules. Not surprisingly, many psychopaths are criminals, but many others remain out of prison, using their charm and chameleonlike abilities to cut a wide swath through society and leaving a wake of ruined lives behind them.

Together, these pieces of the puzzle form an image of a self-centered, callous, and remorseless person profoundly lacking in empathy and the ability to form warm emotional relationships with others, a person who functions without the restraints of conscience. If you think about it, you will realize that what is missing in this picture are the very qualities that allow human beings to live in social harmony.

It is not a pretty picture, and some express doubt that such people exist. To dispel this doubt you need only consider the more dramatic examples of psychopathy that have been increasing in our society in recent years. Dozens of books, movies, and television programs, and hundreds of newspaper articles and headlines, tell the story: Psychopaths make up a significant portion of the people the media describe—serial killers, rapists, thieves, swindlers, con men, wife beaters, white-collar criminals, hype-prone stock promoters and "boiler-room" operators, child abusers, gang members, disbarred lawyers, drug barons, professional gamblers, members of organized crime, doctors who've lost their licenses, terrorists, cult leaders, mercenaries, and unscrupulous businesspeople.

Read the newspaper in this light, and the clues to the extent of the problem virtually jump off the page. Most dramatic are the cold-blooded, conscienceless killers who both repel and fascinate the public. Consider this small sampling from the hundreds of accounts available, many of which have been made into movies:

- John Gacy, a Des Plaines, Illinois, contractor and Junior Chamber of Commerce "Man of the Year" who entertained children as "Pogo the Clown," had his picture taken with President Carter's wife, Rosalynn, and murdered thirty-two young men in the 1970s, burying most of the bodies in the crawl space under his house.[1]

- Charles Sobhraj, a French citizen born in Saigon who was described by his father as a "destructor," became an international confidence man, smuggler, gambler, and murderer who left a trail of empty wallets, bewildered women, drugged tourists, and dead bodies across much of Southeast Asia in the 1970s.[2]

- Jeffrey MacDonald, a physician with the Green Berets who murdered his wife and two children in 1970, claimed that "acid heads" had committed the crimes, became the focus of a great deal of media attention, and was the subject of the book and movie *Fatal Vision*.[3]

- Gary Tison, a convicted murderer who masterfully manipulated the criminal justice system, used his three sons to help him escape from an Arizona prison in 1978, and went on a vicious killing spree that took the lives of six people.[4]

- Kenneth Bianchi, one of the "Hillside Stranglers" who raped, tortured, and murdered a dozen women in the Los

3

Angeles area in the late 1970s, turned in his cousin and accomplice (Angelo Buono), and fooled some experts into believing that he was a multiple personality and that the crimes had been committed by "Steve."[5]

- Richard Ramirez, a Satan-worshipping serial killer known as the "Night Stalker," who proudly described himself as "evil," was convicted in 1987 of thirteen murders and thirty other felonies, including robbery, burglary, rape, sodomy, oral copulation, and attempted murder.[6]

- Diane Downs, who shot her own children to attract a man who didn't want children, and portrayed herself as the real victim.[7]

- Ted Bundy, the "All-American" serial killer who was responsible for the murders of several dozen young women in the mid-1970s, claimed that he had read too much pornography and that a "malignant entity" had taken over his consciousness, and was recently executed in Florida.[8]

- Clifford Olson, a Canadian serial murderer who persuaded the government to pay him $100,000 to show the authorities where he buried his young victims, does everything he can to remain in the spotlight.[9]

- Joe Hunt, a fast-talking manipulator who masterminded a rich-kids' phony investment scheme (popularly known as the Billionaire Boys Club) in Los Angeles in the early 1980s, conned wealthy people into parting with their money, and was involved in two murders.[10]

- William Bradfield, a smooth-talking classics teacher convicted of killing a colleague and her two children.[11]

- Ken McElroy, who for years "robbed, raped, burned, shot . . . and maimed the citizens of Skidmore, Missouri, without conscience or remorse" until he was finally shot dead in 1981 as forty-five people watched.[12]

- Colin Pitchfork, an English "flasher," rapist, and murderer, was the first killer to be convicted on the basis of DNA evidence.[13]

- Kenneth Taylor, a philandering New Jersey dentist who abandoned his first wife, tried to kill his second wife, savagely beat his third wife on their honeymoon in 1983, battered her to death the next year, hid her body in the trunk of his car while he visited his parents and his second wife, and later claimed he had killed his wife in self-defense when she attacked him following his "discovery" that she was sexually abusing their infant child.[14]

- Constantine Paspalakis and Deidre Hunt, who videotaped their torture and murder of a young man, are now on death row.[15]

Individuals of this sort, and the terrifying crimes they commit, certainly grab our attention. Sometimes they share the spotlight with a mixed bag of killers and mass murderers whose crimes, often unbelievably horrific, appear to be related to serious mental problems—for example, Ed Gein, a psychotic killer who skinned and ate his victims;[16] Edmund Kemper, the "co-ed killer," sexual sadist, and necrophiliac who mutilated and dismembered his victims;[17] David Berkowitz, the "Son of Sam" killer who preyed on young couples in parked cars;[18] and Jeffrey Dahmer, the "Milwaukee monster" who pleaded guilty to torturing, killing, and mutilating fifteen men and boys, and was sentenced to fifteen consecutive life terms.[19] Although these killers often judged sane—as were Kemper, Berkowitz, and Dahmer—their unspeakable acts, their grotesque sexual fantasies, and their fascination with power, torture, and death severely test the bounds of sanity.

Psychopathic killers, however, are not mad, according to accepted legal and psychiatric standards. Their acts result not from a deranged mind but from a cold, calculating rationality combined with a chilling inability to treat others as thinking, feeling human beings. Such morally incomprehensible behavior, exhibited by a seemingly normal person, leaves us feeling bewildered and helpless.

As disturbing as this is, we must be careful to keep some perspective here, for the fact is that the majority of psychopaths manage to ply their trade without murdering people. By focusing too much on the most brutal and newsworthy examples of their behavior, we run the risk of remaining blind to the larger picture: psychopaths who don't kill but who have a personal impact on our daily lives. We are far more likely to lose our life savings to an oily-tongued swindler than our lives to a steely-eyed killer.

Nevertheless, high-profile cases have considerable value. Typically they are well documented, alerting us to the fact that such people exist, and that before being caught they were relatives, neighbors, or co-workers of people just like us. These examples also illustrate a frightful and perplexing theme that runs through the case histories of all psychopaths: a deeply disturbing inability to care about the pain and suffering experienced by others—in short, a complete lack of empathy, the prerequisite for love.

In a desperate attempt to explain this lack, we turn first to family background, but there is little to help us there. It is true that the childhoods of *some* psychopaths were characterized by material and emotional deprivation and physical abuse, but for every adult psychopath from a troubled background there is another whose family life apparently was warm and nurturing, and whose siblings are normal, conscientious people with the ability to care deeply for others. Furthermore, most people who had horrible childhoods do not become psychopaths or callous killers. Illuminating as they may be in other areas of human development, the arguments that children subjected to abuse and violence become abusive and violent adults are of limited value here. There are deeper, more elusive explanations of why and how psychopathy emerges. This book represents my quarter-century search for those answers.

A major part of this quest has been a concerted effort to develop an accurate means by which to identify psychopaths among us. For, if we can't spot them, we are doomed to be their victims, both as individuals and as a society. To give just one, all-too-common example, most people are perplexed whenever a convicted killer, paroled from prison, promptly commits another violent offense. They ask incredulously, "Why was such a person released?" Their puzzlement would no doubt turn to outrage if they knew that in many cases the offender was a psychopath whose violent recidivism could have been predicted if the authorities—including the parole board—had only done their homework. It is my hope that this book will help the general public and the criminal justice system to become more aware of the nature of psychopathy, the enormity of the problems it poses, and the steps that can be taken to reduce its devastating impact on our lives.

Chapter 1

"Experiencing" the Psychopath

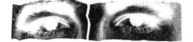

> I could see the dark blood from Halmea's mouth trickling down the sheet toward the part of her that was under Hud. I didn't move or blink, but then Hud was standing up grinning at me; he was buckling his ruby belt buckle. "Ain't she a sweet patootie?" he said. He whistled and began to tuck his pant legs into the tops of his red suede boots. Halmea had curled toward the wall. . . .
> —Larry McMurty, *Horseman, Pass By*

Over the years I've become accustomed to the following experience. In response to a courteous question by a dinner acquaintance about my work, I briefly sketch the distinguishing characteristics of a psychopath. Invariably, someone at the table suddenly looks thoughtful and then exclaims, "Good lord—I think So-and-So must have been . . ." or, "You know, I never realized it before, but the person you're describing is my brother-in-law."

These thoughtful, troubled responses aren't limited to the social realm. Routinely, people who have read of my work call my laboratory to describe a husband, a child, an employer, or an acquaintance whose inexplicable behavior has been causing them grief and pain for years.

8

Nothing is more convincing of the need for clarity and reflection on psychopathy than these real-life stories of disappointment and despair. The three that make up this chapter provide a way of easing into this strange and fascinating subject by conveying that characteristic sense that "something's wrong here but I can't quite put my finger on it."

One of the accounts is drawn from a prison population, where most of the studies of psychopathy take place (for the practical reasons that there are a lot of psychopaths in prisons and the information needed to diagnose them is readily available).

The two other accounts are drawn from everyday life, for psychopaths are found not only in prison populations. Parents, children, spouses, lovers, co-workers, and unlucky victims everywhere are at this moment attempting to cope with the personal chaos and confusion psychopaths cause and to understand what drives them. Many of you will find an uneasy resemblance between the individuals in these examples and people who have made you think you were living in hell.

Ray

After I received my master's degree in psychology in the early 1960s, I looked for a job to help support my wife and infant daughter and to pay for the next stage of my education. Without having been inside a prison before, I found myself employed as the sole psychologist at the British Columbia Penitentiary.

I had no practical work experience as a psychologist and no particular interest in clinical psychology or criminological issues. The maximum-security penitentiary near Vancouver was a formidable institution housing the kinds of criminals I had only heard about through the media. To say I was on unfamiliar ground is an understatement.

I started work completely cold—with no training program or sage mentor to hint at how one went about being a prison psychologist. On the first day I met the warden and his administrative staff, all of whom wore uniforms and some of whom wore sidearms. The prison was run along military lines, and accordingly I was expected to wear a "uniform" consisting of a blue blazer, gray flannel trousers, and black shoes. I convinced the warden that the outfit was unnecessary, but he nevertheless insisted that one at least be made for me by the prison shop, and I was sent down to be measured.

The result was an early sign that all was not as orderly as the place appeared: The jacket sleeves were far too short, the trousers legs were of hilariously discrepant length, and the shoes differed from each other by two sizes. I found the latter particularly perplexing, because the inmate who had measured my feet had been extremely meticulous in tracing them out on a sheet of brown paper. How he could have produced two entirely different-sized shoes, even after several complaints on my part, was difficult to imagine. I could only assume that he was giving me a message of some sort.

My first workday was quite eventful. I was shown to my office, an immense area on the top floor of the prison, far different from the intimate, trust-inspiring burrow I had hoped for. I was isolated from the rest of the institution and had to pass through several sets of locked doors to reach my office. On the wall above my desk was a highly conspicuous red button. A guard who had no idea what a psychologist was supposed to do in a prison—an ignorance I shared—told me that the button was for an emergency, but that if I ever need to press it, I should not expect help to arrive immediately.

The psychologist who was my predecessor had left a small library in the office. It consisted mainly of books on psychological tests, such as the Rorschach Ink Blot Test and the Thematic Apperception Test. I knew something about such tests but had never used them, so the books—among the few objects in the prison that seemed familiar—only reinforced my sense that I was in for a difficult time.

I wasn't in my office for more than an hour when my first "client" arrived. He was a tall, slim, dark-haired man in his thirties. The air around him seemed to buzz, and the eye contact he made with me was so direct and intense that I wondered if I had ever really looked anybody in the eye before. That stare was unrelenting—he didn't indulge in the brief glances away that most people use to soften the force of their gaze.

Without waiting for an introduction, the inmate—I'll call him

Ray—opened the conversation: "Hey, Doc, how's it going? Look, I've got a problem. I need your help. I'd really like to talk to you about this."

Eager to begin work as a genuine psychotherapist, I asked him to tell me about it. In response, he pulled out a knife and waved it in front of my nose, all the while smiling and maintaining that intense eye contact. My first thought was to push the red button behind me, which was in Ray's plain view and the purpose of which was unmistakable. Perhaps because I sensed that he was only testing me, or perhaps because I knew that pushing the button would do no good if he really intended to harm me, I refrained.

Once he determined that I wasn't going to push the button, he explained that he intended to use the knife not on me but on another inmate who had been making overtures to his "protégé," a prison term for the more passive member of a homosexual pairing. Just why he was telling me this was not immediately clear, but I soon suspected that he was checking me out, trying to determine what sort of a prison employee I was. If I said nothing about the incident to the administration, I would be violating a strict prison rule that required staff to report possession of a weapon of any sort. On the other hand, I knew that if I did report him, word would get around that I was not an inmate-oriented psychologist, and my job would be even more difficult than it was promising to be. Following our session, in which he described his "problem" not once or twice but many times, I kept quiet about the knife. To my relief, he didn't stab the other inmate, but it soon became evident that Ray had caught me in his trap: I had shown myself to be a soft touch who would overlook clear violations of fundamental prison rules in order to develop "professional" rapport with the inmates.

From that first meeting on, Ray managed to make my eight-month stint at the prison miserable. His constant demands on my time and his attempts to manipulate me into doing things for him were unending. On one occasion, he convinced me that he would make a good cook—he felt he had a natural bent for cooking, he thought he would become a chef when he was released, this was a great opportunity to try out some of his ideas to make institutional food preparation more efficient, etc.—and I supported his request for a transfer from the machine shop (where he had apparently made the knife). What I didn't consider was that the kitchen was a source of sugar, potatoes, fruit, and other ingredients that could be turned into alcohol. Several months after I had recommended the transfer, there was a mighty eruption below the floorboards directly under the warden's table. When the commotion died down, we found an elaborate system for distilling alcohol below the floor. Something had gone wrong and one of the pots had exploded. There was nothing unusual about the presence of a still in a maximum-security prison, but the audacity of placing one under the warden's seat shook up a lot of people. When it was discovered that Ray was brains behind the bootleg operation, he spent some time in solitary confinement.

Once out of "the hole," Ray appeared in my office as if nothing had happened and asked for a transfer from the kitchen to the auto shop—he really felt he had a knack, he saw the need to prepare himself for the outside world, if he only had the time to practice he could have his own body shop on the outside . . . . I was still feeling the sting of having arranged the first transfer, but eventually he wore me down.

Soon afterward I decided to leave the prison to pursue a Ph.D. in psychology, and about a month before I left Ray almost persuaded me to ask my father, a roofing contractor, to offer him a job as part of an application for parole. When I mentioned this to some of the prison staff, they found it hard to stop laughing. They knew Ray well, they'd all been taken in by his schemes and plans for reform, and one by one they had resolved to adopt a skeptical approach to him. Jaded? I thought so at the time. But the fact was that their picture of Ray was clearer than mine—despite my job description. Theirs had been brought into focus by years of experience with people like him.

Ray had an incredible ability to con not just me but everybody. He could talk, and lie, with a smoothness and a directness that sometimes momentarily disarmed even the most experienced and cynical of the prison staff. When I met him he had a long criminal record behind him (and, as it turned out, ahead of him); about half his adult life had been spent in prison, and many of his crimes had been violent. Yet he convinced me, and others more experienced than I, of his readiness to reform, that his interest in crime had been completely overshadowed by a driving passion in—well, cooking, mechanics, you name it. He lied endlessly, lazily, about everything, and it disturbed him not a whit whenever I pointed out something in his file that contradicted one of his lies. He would simply change the subject and spin off in a different direction. Finally convinced that he might not make the perfect job candidate in my father's firm, I turned down Ray's request—and was shaken by his nastiness at my refusal.

Before I left the prison for the university, I was still making payments on a 1958 Ford that I could not really afford. One of the officers there, later to become warden, offered to trade his 1950 Morris Minor for my Ford and to take over my payments. I agreed, and because the Morris wasn't in very good shape I took advantage of the prison policy of letting staff have their cars repaired in the institution's auto shop—where Ray still worked, thanks (he would have said no thanks) to me. The car received a beautiful paint job and the motor and drivetrain were reconditioned.

With all our possessions on top of the car and our baby in a plywood bed in the backseat, my wife and I headed for Ontario. The first problems appeared soon after we left Vancouver, when the motor seemed a bit rough. Later, when we encountered some moderate inclines, the radiator boiled over. A garage mechanic discovered ball bearings in the carburetor's float chamber; he also pointed out where one of the hoses to the radiator had clearly been tampered with. These problems were repaired easily enough, but the next one, which arose while we were going down a long hill, was more serious. The brake pedal became very spongy and then simply dropped to the floor—no brakes, and it was a *long* hill. Fortunately, we made it to a service station, where we found that the brake line had been cut so that a slow leak would occur. Perhaps it was a coincidence that Ray was working in the auto shop when the car was being tuned up, but I had no doubt that the prison "telegraph" had informed him of the new owner of the car.

At the university, I prepared to write my dissertation on the effects of punishment on human learning and performance. In my research for the project I encountered for the first time the literature on psychopathy. I'm not sure I thought of Ray at the time, but circumstances conspired to bring him to mind.

My first job after receiving my Ph.D. was at the University of British Columbia, not far from the penitentiary where I had worked several years before. During registration week in that precomputer age, I sat behind a table with several colleagues to register long lines of students for their fall classes. As I was dealing with a student my ears pricked up at the mention of my name. "Yes, I worked as Dr. Hare's assistant at the penitentiary the whole time he was there, a year or so, I would say it was. Did all his paperwork for him, filled him in on prison life. Sure, he used to talk over hard cases with me. We worked great together." It was Ray, standing at the head of the next line.

My *assistant!* I broke into the easy flow of his remarks with, "Oh, really?" expecting to disconcert him. "Hey, Doc, how's it going?" he called without losing a beat. Then he simply jumped back into his conversation and took off in another direction. Later, when I checked his application forms, it became apparent that his transcript of previous university courses was fraudulent. To his credit, he had not attempted to register in one of *my* courses.

Perhaps what fascinated me most was that Ray remained absolutely unflappable even *after* his deceit was revealed—and that my colleague was clearly going along for the ride. What, in his psychological makeup, gave Ray the power to override reality, apparently without compunction or concern? As it turned out, I would spend the next twenty-five years doing empirical research to answer that question.

The story of Ray has its amusing side now, after so many years. Less amusing are the case studies of the hundreds of psychopaths that I have studied since then.

I HAD BEEN at the prison for a few months when the administration sent an inmate to me for psychological testing prior to a parole hearing. He was serving a six-year sentence for manslaughter. When I realized that the complete report of the offense was missing from my files, I asked him to fill me in on the details. The inmate said that his girlfriend's infant daughter had been crying nonstop for hours and because she smelled he reluctantly decided to change her diapers. "She shit all over my hand and I lost my temper," he said, a grisly euphemism for what he really did. "I picked her up by the feet and smashed her against the wall," he said with—unbelievably—a smile on his face. I was stunned by the casual description of his appalling behavior, and, thinking about my own infant daughter, I unprofessionally kicked him out of my office and refused to see him again.

Curious about what subsequently happened to this man, I recently tracked down his prison files. I learned that he had received parole a year after I had left the prison, and that he had been killed during a high-speed police chase following a bungled bank robbery. The prison psychiatrist had diagnosed this man as a psychopath and had recommended against parole. The parole board could not really be faulted for having ignored this professional advice. At the time, the procedures for the diagnosis of psychopathy were vague and unreliable, and the implications of such a diagnosis for the prediction of behavior were not yet known. As we will see, the situation is quite different now, and any parole board whose decision does not take into account current knowledge about psychopathy and recidivism runs the risk of making a potentially disastrous mistake.

Elsa and Dan

She met him in a laundromat in London, where she was taking a year off from teaching after a stormy and exhausting divorce. She'd seen him around the neighborhood, and when they finally started to talk she felt as if she knew him. He was open and friendly and they hit it off right away. From the start she thought he was hilarious.

She'd been lonely. The weather was grim and sleety, she'd already seen every movie and play in the city, and she didn't know a soul east of the Atlantic.

"Ah, traveler's loneliness," Dan crooned sympathetically over dinner. "It's the worst."

15

After dessert he was embarrassed to discover he'd come out without his wallet. Elsa was more than happy to pay for dinner, more than happy to sit through the double feature she had seen earlier in the week. At the pub, over drinks, he told her he was a translator for the United Nations. He traveled the globe. He was, at the moment, between assignments.

They saw each other four times that week, five the week after. Dan lived in a flat at the top of a house somewhere in Hampstead, he told her, but it wasn't long before he had all but moved in with Elsa. To her amazement, she loved the arrangement. It was against her nature, she wasn't even sure how it had happened, but after her long stint of loneliness she was having the time of her life.

Still, there were details, unexplained, undiscussed, that she shoved out of her mind. He never invited her to his home; she never met his friends. One night he brought over a carton filled with tape recorders—plastic-wrapped straight from the factory, unopened; a few days later they were gone. Once Elsa came home to find three televisions stacked in the corner. "Storing them for a friend," was all he told her. When she pressed for more, he merely shrugged.

The first time Dan failed to show up at a prearranged place, she was frantic that he'd been hurt in traffic—he was always darting across the street in the middle of the block.

He stayed away for three days and was asleep on the bed when she came home in midmorning. The odor of rancid perfume and stale beer nearly made her sick, and her fear for his life was replaced with something new for her: awful, wild, uncontrollable jealousy. "Where have you *been?*" she cried. "I've been so worried. Where *were* you?"

He looked sour as he woke up. "Don't ever ask me that," he snapped. "I won't have it."

"What—?"

"Where I go, what I do, who I do it with—it doesn't concern you, Elsa. Don't ask."

He was like a different person. But then he seemed to pull himself together, shook the sleep off, and reached out to her. "I know it hurts you," he said in his old gentle way, "but think of jealousy as a flu, and wait to get over it. And you will, baby, you will." Like a mother cat licking her kitten, he groomed her back into trusting him. And yet she thought what he'd said about jealousy was so odd. It made her sure that he had never felt anything like the pain of a broken trust.

One night she asked him lightly if he felt like stepping out to the corner and bringing her an ice cream. He didn't reply, and when she glanced up she found him glaring at her furiously. "Always got everything you wanted, didn't you," he said in a strange, snide way. "Any little thing little Elsa wanted, somebody always jumped up and ran out and bought it for her, didn't they?"

"Are you kidding? I'm not like that. What are you talking about?"

He got up from the chair and walked out. She never saw him again.

The Twins

On their twin daughters' thirtieth birthday, Helen and Steve looked back with mixed feelings. Every burst of pride in Ariel's accomplishments was cut short by an awful memory of Alice's unpredictable, usually destructive, and often expensive behavior. They were fraternal twins but had always borne a striking physical resemblance to each other; however, in personality they differed like day and night—perhaps the more appropriate metaphor was heaven and hell.

If anything, the contrast had grown starker over three decades. Ariel had called last week to share great news—the senior partners had made it clear to her that if she continued as she was, she surely would be invited to join their ranks in four or five years. The call from Alice—or rather Alice's floor counselor—was not so cheerful. Alice and another resident at the halfway house had left in the middle of the night and hadn't been seen in two days. The last time this had happened, Alice had surfaced in Alaska, hungry and penniless. By then, her parents had lost count of how many times they had wired money and arranged for Alice to fly home.

While Ariel had had her share of problems growing up, they

had always been more or less normal. She had been moody and sullen when she didn't get her way, even more so during adolescence. She had tried cigarettes and marijuana in her junior year in high school; she had dropped out of college in her sophomore year, fearing that her lack of direction meant that she lacked potential. During that year in the work force, though, Ariel decided on law school, and from that point on nothing could stop her. She was focused, fascinated, and ambitious. She made Law Review in school, graduated with honors, and landed the job she went after in her first interview.

With Alice, there had always been "something a little *off.*" Both girls were little beauties, but Helen was amazed to see that even at age three or four Alice knew how to use her looks and her little-girl cuteness to get her way. Helen even felt that somehow Alice knew how to flirt—she put on all her airs when there were men around—even though having such thoughts about her young daughter made her feel terribly guilty. Helen felt even guiltier when a small kitten given to the girls by a cousin was found dead, strangled, in the yard. Ariel clearly was heartbroken; Alice's tears seemed a little forced. Much as she tried to banish the thought, Helen felt that Alice had had something to do with the kitten's death.

Sisters fight, but again, "something was off," in the way these twins went at it. Ariel was *always* on the defensive; Alice was *always* the aggressor, and she seemed to take special pleasure in ruining her sister's things. It was a great relief to everybody when Alice left home at age seventeen—at least Ariel could now live in peace. It soon became clear, however, that upon moving out of the house Alice had discovered drugs. Now she was not only unpredictable, impulsive, and liable to throw fierce tantrums to get her way—she had become an addict, and she supported her habit any way she could, including theft and prostitution. Bail and treatment programs—$10,000 for three weeks at one pricey clinic in New Hampshire—became a continual financial drain for Helen and Steve. "I'm glad *somebody* in this family is going to be solvent," Steve said when he heard Ariel's good news. He had been wondering for some time just how much longer he could afford to clean up after Alice. In fact, he had seriously been reconsidering the wisdom of trying to keep her out of prison. After all, wasn't it she, not he and Helen, who should face the consequences of her actions?

Helen was adamant on the subject: No child of hers would spend a single night in prison (Alice had already spent quite a number of them, but Helen chose to forget) as long as she was there to pay bail. It became a question of responsibility: Helen fully believed that she and Steve had done something wrong in bringing up Alice, although in thirty years of intense self-scrutiny she honestly couldn't identify their mistake. Perhaps it was subconscious, though—maybe she hadn't been as enthusiastic as she might have been when the doctor told her he suspected she would have twins. Maybe she had unknowingly slighted Alice, who was heartier than Ariel at birth. Maybe somehow she and Steve had set off the Jekyll and Hyde syndrome by insisting that the girls never dress as twins and go to separate dance schools and summer camps.

Maybe . . . but Helen doubted it. Didn't all parents make mistakes? Didn't all parents inadvertently favor one child over the other, if only temporarily? Didn't all parents feel their delight in their children ebb and flow with the contingencies of life? Yes indeed—but not all parents wound up with an Alice. In her search for answers during the girls' childhood, Helen had observed other families intensely, and she had seen some very careless, very unfair parents blessed with stable, well-adjusted children. She knew that blatantly abusive parents generally produced troubled if not disturbed children, but Helen was sure that for all their mistakes, she and Steve hardly fell into that category.

So, the girls' thirtieth birthday brought Helen and Steve mixed feelings—gratitude that their twins were physically healthy, happiness that Ariel had found security and fulfillment in her work, and the old, familiar anxiety as to Alice's whereabouts and welfare. But perhaps the overriding feeling as this long-married couple drank a toast to their absent daughters' birthday was dismay that after all this time nothing had changed. This was the twentieth century—they were supposed to know how to fix things. There were pills you could take to recover from depression, treatments to control phobias, but not one of the myriad doctors, psychiatrists, psychologists, treatment counselors, and social workers who had seen Alice over the years had come up with an explanation or an antidote for her problem. Nobody was even sure whether she was mentally ill. After thirty years, Helen and Steve looked across the table and asked sadly, "Is she crazy? Or just plain bad?"

Chapter 2

Focusing
the Picture

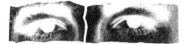

He will choose you, disarm you with his words, and control you with this presence. He will delight you with his wit and his plans. He will show you a good time, but you will always get the bill. He will smile and deceive you, and he will scare you with his eyes. And when he is through with you, and he will be through with you, he will desert you and take with him your innocence and your pride. You will be left much sadder but not a lot wiser, and for a long time you will wonder what happened and what you did wrong. And if another of his kind comes knocking at your door, will you open it?
—From an essay signed, "A psychopath in prison."

The question remains: "Is Alice mad or bad?"

It's a question that has long troubled not just psychologists and psychiatrists but philosophers and theologians. Formally stated, is the psychopath mentally ill or simply a rule breaker who is perfectly aware of what he or she is doing?

This question is not just a semantic one; posed another way, it has immeasurable practical significance: Does the treatment or control of the psychopath rightly fall to mental health professionals or to the correctional system? Everywhere in the world, judges, social workers, lawyers, schoolteachers, mental health workers, doctors, correctional staff, and members of the general public need—whether they know it or not—the answer.

The Ramifications
of the Question

For most people, the confusion and uncertainty surrounding this subject begin with the word *psychopathy* itself. Literally it means "mental illness" (from *psyche*, "mind"; and *pathos*, "disease"), and this is the meaning of the term still found in some dictionaries. The confusion is compounded by the media use of the term as the equivalent of "insane" or "crazy": "The police say a 'psycho' is on the loose," or, "The guy who killed her must be a 'psycho.' "

Most clinicians and researchers don't use the term in this way; they know that psychopathy cannot be understood in terms of traditional views of mental illness. Psychopaths are not disoriented or out of touch with reality, nor do they experience the delusions, hallucinations, or intense subjective distress that characterize most other mental disorders. Unlike psychotic individuals, psychopaths are rational and aware of what they are doing and why. Their behavior is the result of *choice*, freely exercised.

So, if a person with a diagnosis of schizophrenia breaks society's rules—say, by killing the next passerby in response to orders "received from Martian in a spaceship"—we deem that person not responsible "by reason of insanity." When a person diagnosed as a psychopath breaks the same rules, he or she is judged sane and is sent to prison.

Still, a common response to reports of brutal crimes, particularly serial torture and killing, is: "Anyone would *have* to be crazy to do that." Perhaps so, but not always in the legal or the psychiatric sense of the term.

As I mentioned earlier, some serial killers *are* insane. For example, consider Edward Gein,[1] whose horrific and bizarre crimes became the basis for characters in a number of movies and books, including *Psycho, The Texas Chainsaw Massacre,* and *The Silence of the Lambs.* Gein killed, mutilated, and sometimes ate his victims, and he made grotesque objects—lampshades, clothes, masks—from their body parts and skin. At his trial both prosecution and defense psychiatrists agreed that he was psychotic; the diagnosis was chronic schizophrenia, and the judge committed him to a hospital for the criminally insane.

Most serial killers are not like Gein, however. They may torture, kill, and mutilate their victims—appalling behavior that sorely tests our ideas of what "sanity" means—but in most cases there is no evidence that they are deranged, mentally confused, or psychotic. Many of these killers—Ted Bundy, John Wayne Gacy, Henry Lee Lucas, to name but a few—have been diagnosed as psychopaths, which means they were sane by current psychiatric and legal standards. They were sent to prison and, in some cases, executed. But the distinction between mentally ill killers and sane but psychopathic murderers was by no means easy to come by. It resulted from a centuries-long scientific debate that at times bordered on the metaphysical.

Some Terminology

Many researchers, clinicians, and writers use the terms *psychopath* and *sociopath* interchangeably. For example, in his book *The Silence of the Lambs,* Thomas Harris described Hannibal Lecter as a "pure sociopath," whereas the writer of the movie version called him a "pure psychopath."

Sometimes the term *sociopathy* is used because it is less likely than is *psychopathy* to be confused with psychoticism or insanity. In his book *The Blooding,* Joseph Wambaugh says of Colin Pitchfork, an English rapist-murderer, ". . . it was a pity that the psychiatrist didn't choose to describe him as a 'sociopath' instead of a 'psychopath' in his report, because of the misunderstanding that accompanies the latter. Everyone connected with the case seemed to confuse the word [psychopath] with 'psychotic.' "

In many cases the choice of term reflects the user's views on the *origins and determinants* of the clinical syndrome or disorder described in this book. Thus, some clinicians and researchers—as well as most sociologists and criminologists—who believe that the syndrome is forged entirely by social forces and early experiences prefer the term *socio*path, whereas those—including this writer—who feel that psychological, biological, and genetic factors also contribute to development of the syndrome generally use the term *psycho*path. The same individual therefore could be diagnosed as a sociopath by one expert and as a psychopath by another.

Consider the following exchange between an offender (O) and one of my graduate students (S):

S: "Did you get any feedback from the prison psychiatrist who assessed you?"

O: "She told me I was a . . . not a sociopath . . . a psychopath. This was comical. She said not to worry about it because you can have a doctor or lawyer who is a psychopath. I said, 'Yeah, I understand that. If you were sitting on a plane that was hijacked would you rather be sitting next to me or some sociopath or neurotic who shits his pants and gets us all killed?' She just about fell off her chair. If someone wants to diagnose me I'd rather be a psychopath than a sociopath.' "

S: "Aren't they the same thing?"

O: "No, they're not. You see, a sociopath misbehaves because he's been brought up wrong. Maybe he's got a beef with society. I've got no beef with society. I'm not harboring hostility. It's just the way I am. Yeah, I guess I'd be a psychopath."

A term that was *supposed* to have much the same meaning as "psychopath" or "sociopath" is *antisocial personality disorder*, described in the third edition of the American Psychiatric Association's *Diagnostic and Statistical Manual of Mental Disorders* (DSM-III; 1980) and its revision (DSM-III-R; 1987), widely used as the "diagnostic bible" for mental illness.[2] The diagnostic criteria for antisocial personality disorder consist primarily of a long list of antisocial and criminal behaviors. When the list first appeared it was felt that the average clinician could not reliably assess personality traits such as empathy, egocentricity, guilt, and so forth. Diagnosis therefore was based on what clinicians presumably *could* assess without difficulty, namely objective, socially deviant behaviors.

The result has been confusion during the past decade, with many clinicians mistakenly assuming that antisocial personality disorder and psychopathy are synonymous terms. As diagnosed by the DSM-III and the DSM-III-R, as well as by the recently published DSM-IV (1994), "antisocial personality disorder" refers primarily to a cluster of criminal and antisocial behaviors. The majority of criminals easily meet the criteria for such a diagnosis. "Psychopathy," on the other hand, is defined by a cluster of both personality traits and socially deviant behaviors. Most criminals are *not* psychopaths, and many of the individuals who manage to operate on the shady side of the law and remain out of prison *are* psychopaths. Keep this in mind if you have occasion to consult a clinician or counselor about a psychopath in your life. Make sure that he or she knows the difference between antisocial personality disorder and psychopathy.[3]

A Historical View

One of the first clinicians to write about psychopaths was Philippe Pinel, an early nineteenth-century French psychiatrist. He used the term *insanity without delirium* to describe a pattern of behavior marked by utter remorselessness and a complete lack of restraint, a pattern he considered distinct from the ordinary "evil that men do."[4]

Pinel regarded this condition morally neutral, but other writers considered these patients "morally insane," the very embodiment of evil. So began an argument that spanned generations and that seesawed between the view that psychopaths were "mad" and that they were "bad" or even diabolical.

THE DIRTY DOZEN is a classic movie that glorifies a long-standing Hollywood myth: Turn a psychopath inside out and you find a hero. The plot of the movie concerns a choice given to a handful of the roughest, toughest criminals: volunteer for what amounts to a suicide mission, or stay in prison. The task involves the capture of a castle in which the elite command of the German army is ensconced. Needless to say, the Dirty Dozen succeed in the capture. And needless to say, they are honored as heroes, to the apparent gratification of several generations of audiences.

Psychiatrist James Weiss, author of *All But Me and Thee,* tells a very different tale. His book recounts an investigation conducted during World War II by Brigadier General Elliot D. Cook and his assistant, Colonel Ralph Bing. They started at the end point—the Army East Coast Processing (Detention) Center at Camp Edwards on Cape Cod—and worked backward to company level to determine how the more than two thousand inmates had wound up there.

The story, as Weiss remarks, was "the same sad tale" told over and over again. Knowing the company was going into a fight, the soldier volunteered to go back for supplies and was never heard from again. Or the soldier went from stealing food to stealing a truck, and totaling it on a joyride. Completely unresponsive to interests of their fellow GIs and more attuned to instant gratification than to the fundamental rules of caution in combat, these fellows had a much greater chance of getting shot—"Peterson ... stuck his head up when everyone else had theirs down and a German sniper put a bullet through the middle of it"—than of accomplishing an act of heroism that involved planning, cunning, and actions rooted in conscience.

The Dirty Dozen might look squeaky clean by the time Hollywood gets through with them, but in real life, as Weiss concludes, "conversion by combat seldom if ever happens." (James Weiss, *Journal of Operational Psychiatry* 5, 1974, 119.)

World War II gave the debate a new, practical urgency—more than speculation was necessary. First, with the military draft, the need became pressing to identify, diagnose, and if possible treat individuals who could disrupt or even destroy strict military control, and this issue drew lively public attention. But an even more ominous significance arose with the revelation of the Nazis' machinery of destruction and their cold-blooded program of extermination. What were the dynamics of such a development? How and why could individuals—even, terrifyingly, one individual in command of a nation—operate outside the rules that most people accepted as restraints on their basest impulses and fantasies?

Many writers took up the challenge, but none had as great an impact as Hervey Cleckley. In his now classic book, *The Mask of Sanity,* first published in 1941,[5] Cleckley pleaded for attention to what he recognized as a dire but ignored social problem. He wrote dramatically about his patients and provided the general public with the first detailed view of psychopathy. For example, in his book he included his case notes on Gregory, a young man with a yards-long arrest sheet who had failed to kill his mother only because of a malfunctioning gun.

> It would be impossible to describe adequately this young man's career without writing hundreds of pages. His repeated antisocial acts and the triviality of his apparent motivation as well as his inability to learn by experience to make a better adjustment and avoid serious trouble that can be readily foreseen, all make me feel that he is a classic example of psychopathic personality. I think it very likely that he will continue to behave as he has behaved in the past, and I do not know of any psychiatric treatment that is likely to influence this behavior appreciably or to help him make a better adjustment. (pp. 173–74)

Phrases such as "shrewdness and agility of mind," "talks entertainingly," and "exceptional charm" dot Cleckley's case histories. He noted that a psychopath in jail or prison would use his considerable social skills to persuade a judge that he actually belonged in a mental hospital. Once in the hospital, where nobody wanted him—because he was too disruptive—he would apply his skills to obtaining a release.

Interspersed in his vivid clinical descriptions are Cleckley's own meditations on the meaning of the psychopath's behavior.

> The [psychopath] is unfamiliar with the primary facts or data of what might be called personal values and is altogether incapable of understanding such matters. It is impossible for him to take even a slight interest in the tragedy or joy or the striving of humanity as presented in serious liter-

ature or art. He is also indifferent to all these matters in life itself. Beauty and ugliness, except in a very superficial sense, goodness, evil, love, horror, and humor have no actual meaning, no power to move him. He is, furthermore, lacking in the ability to see that others are moved. It is as though he were color-blind, despite his sharp intelligence, to this aspect of human existence. It cannot be explained to him because there is nothing in his orbit of awareness that can bridge the gap with comparison. He can repeat the words and say glibly that he understands, and there is no way for him to realize that he does not understand (p. 90)

The Mask of Sanity greatly influenced researchers in the United States and Canada and is the clinical framework for much of the scientific research on psychopathy conducted in the past quarter-century. For the most part, the goal of this research has been to find out what makes the psychopath "tick." We now have some important clues, which are described throughout this book. But as our knowledge of the devastation caused by psychopaths at large in society increases, modern research has an even more vital goal—*the development of reliable ways to identify these individuals in order to minimize the risk they pose to others.* This task is of immense importance to the general public and individuals alike. My role in the search began in the 1960s at the psychology department of the University of British Columbia. There, my growing interest in psychopathy merged with my prison experience to form what was to become my life work. Where once I had worked I managed to continue my research.

Identifying "True Psychopaths"

A problem in doing research in prisons is that the inmates generally are suspicious and mistrustful of outsiders, particularly academics. I was helped by an inmate at the top of the prison hierarchy who concluded that my research would have no negative consequences for those who participated and that it might even be of some use in understanding criminal behavior. This inmate, a professional bank robber, became my spokesman, endorsing my work and spreading the word that he himself was a willing participant. The result was a great surge of volunteers, an embarrassment of riches that brought with it its own problem: How was I to distinguish the "true" psychopaths from the rest of the volunteers?

In the 1960s psychologists and psychiatrists were by no means in complete agreement on what distinguished the psychopath. The problem of classification was a major stumbling block. We were attempting to sort human beings, not apples and oranges, and the distinguishing features we were concerned with were psychological phenomena, well hidden from the probing eye of science.

A WOMAN IN Florida bought him a new car.

A woman in California bought him a motor home.

Who knows who else bought him what else.

As a newspaper article describing Leslie Gall's cross country exploits aptly pointed out, it's all in the name: Gall says it all.

The "sweetheart swindler," as one of his victims referred to him, made his way from widow to widow, bilking them out of all he needed and far more. They opened their hearts and their checkbooks to him. "With nerve, charm, and a suitcase full of false IDs, he allegedly stole tens of thousands of dollars from elderly women he met at senior citizens' dances and social clubs. In looking into his background, California police found a lengthy criminal record, all related to fraud, forgery, and theft.

When Gall learned that the California police were on his trail, he had his lawyer write a letter to police in Florida saying that he was willing to turn himself in in exchange for a guarantee that he could do his time in a Canadian prison.

"Since the story was made public," wrote reporter Dale Brazao, California police phones were "ringing constantly with calls from people saying they think Gall may have also been involved with their mother or an aunt. 'He's got that I-think-I-know-that-guy kind of a face. . . . Who knows how many more victims will come forward."

Now serving a ten-year sentence in a Florida prison, Gall

portrays himself as a humanitarian. "Sure I took their money, but they got their money's worth out of me," he said. "I fulfilled their need. They got attention, affection, companionship, and, in some cases, they got love. . . . There were times we didn't even get out of bed." (Based on articles by Dale Brazao, *Toronto Star*, May 19, 1990, and April 20, 1992.)

I might have used standard psychological tests to identify psychopathic inmates, but most of those tests depended on self-reporting—for example, "I lie (1) easily; (2) with some difficulty; (3) never." The inmate population I was working with was quite adept at figuring out what psychiatrists and psychologists were trying to get at when they used tests and interviews. Generally, they saw no reason to reveal anything of real significance to prison staff members but every reason to show themselves to the best advantage with respect to possible parole, change of work assignment, admission to some program or other, and so forth. Moreover, the psychopaths among them were expert at distorting and molding the truth to suit their purposes. Impression management was definitely one of their strong suits.

As a result, the prison records were often filled with carefully written personality profiles that seemed embarrassingly at odds with what everyone else in the prison knew about the inmates in question. I recall one file in which the psychologist had used a battery of self-report tests to conclude that a callous killer was actually a sensitive, caring individual who needed only the psychological equivalent of a warm hug! Because of the uncritical use of personality tests, the literature was (and still is) cluttered with studies that purported to be about psychopathy but actually had very little to do with it.

One inmate provided a great example of why I was reluctant to rely on psychological tests. During the course of an interview with him in one of my research projects, the topic of psychological tests came up. He told me that he knew all about them, particularly about the self-report inventory most popular with prison psychologists, the Minnesota Multiphasic Personality Inventory, or MMPI. As it turned out, this fellow had in his cell a complete set of question booklets, scoring sheets, scoring templates, and interpretive manuals for the MMPI. He used this material, and the expertise it gave him, to provide a consulting service for other inmates—for a fee, of course. He would determine what sort of profile his client should have, given his circumstances and objectives, and then coach him on how to answer the questions.

"Just arrived in the prison? What you want to show is that you're a bit disturbed, perhaps depressed and anxious, but not disturbed in such a way that you can't be treated. When you're close to a parole date come and see me again, and we'll arrange for you to show significant improvement."

Even without such "professional" help, many criminals are able to fake the results of psychological tests without too much difficulty. Recently, an inmate in one of my research projects had an institutional file that contained three completely different MMPI profiles. Obtained about a year apart, the first suggested that the man was psychotic, the second that he was perfectly normal, and the third that he was mildly disturbed. During our interview he offered the opinion that psychologists and psychiatrists were "air heads" who believed anything he told them. He said he had faked mental illness on the first test in order to receive a transfer to the psychiatric unit of the prison, where he thought he could do "easy time." On finding that the unit was not to his liking ("too many buggy cons") he managed to take another MMPI, this time coming out normal, and was moved back to the main prison. Soon afterward, he decided to portray himself as anxious and depressed, and produced an MMPI profile suggestive of mild disturbance, whereupon he was given Valium, which he sold to other inmates. The irony here is that the prison psychologist treated each of the three MMPI profiles as valid indications of the type and degree of psychiatric disturbance suffered by the inmate.

I decided to grapple with the classification problem by not relying solely on self-reporting. To gather my data, I assembled a team of clinicians who were thoroughly familiar with Cleckley's work. They would identify psychopaths for study in the prison population by means of long, detailed interviews and close study of file information. I provided these "raters" with Cleckley's list of the characteristics of psychopathy to serve as a guideline. As it turned out, agreement among the clinicians was generally very high; the few disagreements that arose were resolved by discussion.

Still, other researchers and clinicians were never certain about just *how* we made our diagnoses. Therefore, my students and I spent more than ten years improving and refining our procedures for ferreting the psychopaths out of the general prison population. The result was a highly reliable diagnostic tool that any clinician or researcher could use and that yielded a richly detailed profile of the personality disorder called psychopathy. We named this instrument the *Psychopathy Checklist.*[6] For the first time, a generally accepted, scientifically sound means of measuring and diagnosing psychopathy became available. The *Psychopathy Checklist* is now used worldwide to help clinicians and researchers distinguish with reasonable certainty true psychopaths from those who merely break the rules.

Chapter 3

The Profile: Feelings and Relationships

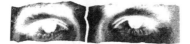

Do I care about other people? That's a tough one. But, yeah, I guess I really do ... but I don't let my feelings get in the way.... I mean, I'm as warm and caring as the next guy, but let's face it, everyone's trying to screw you.... You've got to look out for yourself, park your feelings. Say you need something, or someone messes with you ... maybe tries to rip you off ... you take care of it ... do whatever needs to be done.... Do I feel bad if I have to hurt someone? Yeah, sometimes. But mostly it's like ... uh ... [laughs] ... how did you feel the last time you squashed a bug?
> —A psychopath doing time for kidnapping, rape, and extortion

The *Psychopathy Checklist* lets us discuss psychopaths with little risk that we are describing simple social deviance or criminality, or that we are mislabeling people who have nothing more in common than that they have broken the law. But it also provides a detailed picture of the disordered personalities of the psychopaths among us. In this chapter and the next I bring that picture into focus by describing the more salient features one by one. This chapter looks at the emotional and interpersonal traits of this complex personality disorder; chapter 4 examines the unstable, characteristically antisocial lifestyle of the psychopath.

Key Symptoms of Psychopathy

Emotional/Interpersonal	Social Deviance
• glib and superficial	• impulsive
• egocentric and grandiose	• poor behavior controls
• lack of remorse or guilt	• need for excitement
• lack of empathy	• lack of responsibility
• deceitful and manipulative	• early behavior problems
• shallow emotions	• adult antisocial behavior

A Cautionary Note

The *Psychopathy Checklist* is a complex clinical tool for professional use.[1] What follows is a general summary of the key traits and behaviors of psychopaths. **Do not use these symptoms to diagnose yourself or others.** A diagnosis requires explicit training and access to the formal scoring manual. If you suspect that someone you know conforms to the profile described here and in the next chapter, and if it is important to you to obtain an expert opinion, seek the services of a qualified (registered) forensic psychologist or psychiatrist.

Also, be aware that people who are *not* psychopaths may have *some* of the symptoms described here. Many people are impulsive, or glib, or cold and unfeeling, or antisocial, but this does not mean they are psychopaths. Psychopathy is a *syndrome*—a cluster of related symptoms.

Glib and Superficial

Psychopaths are often witty and articulate. They can be amusing and entertaining conversationalists, ready with a quick and clever comeback, and can tell unlikely but convincing stories that cast themselves in a good light. They can be very effective in presenting themselves well and are often very likable and charming. To some people, however, they seem too slick and smooth, too obviously insincere and superficial. Astute observers often get the impression that psychopaths are play-acting, mechanically "reading their lines."

One of my raters described an interview she did with a prisoner: "I sat down and took out my clipboard, and the first thing this guy told me was what beautiful eyes I had. He managed to work quite a few compliments on my appearance into the interview—couldn't get over my hair. So by the time I wrapped things up I was feeling unusually . . . well, pretty. I'm a wary person, especially on the job, and can usually spot a phony. When I got back outside, I couldn't believe I'd fallen for a line like that."

Psychopaths may ramble and tell stories that seem unlikely in light of what is known about them. Typically, they attempt to appear familiar with sociology, psychiatry, medicine, psychology, philosophy, poetry, literature, art, or law. A signpost to this trait is often a smooth lack of concern at being found out. One of our prison files describes a psychopathic inmate claiming to have advanced degrees in sociology and psychology, when in fact he did not even complete high school. He maintained the fiction during an interview with one of my students, a Ph.D. candidate in psychology; she commented that the inmate was so confident in his use of technical jargon and concepts that those not familiar with the field of psychology might well have been impressed. Variations on this sort of "expert" theme are common among psychopaths.

DICK! SMOOTH. SMART. Yes, you had to hand it to him. Christ, it was incredible how he could "con a guy." Like the clerk in the Kansas City, Missouri, clothing store, the first of the places Dick had decided to "hit." . . . Dick told him, "All I want you to do is stand there. Don't laugh, and don't be surprised at anything I say. You've got to play these things by ear." For the task proposed, it seemed, Dick had the perfect pitch. He breezed in, breezily introduced Perry to the clerk as

35

"a friend of mine about to get married," and went on, "I'm his best man. Helping kind of shop around for the clothes he'll want. . . ." The salesman ate it up, and soon Perry, stripped of his denim trousers, was trying on a gloomy suit the clerk considered "ideal for an informal ceremony." . . . They then selected a gaudy array of jackets and slacks regarded as appropriate for what was to be, according to Dick, a Florida honeymoon. . . . "How about that? An ugly runt like him, he's making it with a honey she's not only built but loaded. While guys like you and me, good-looking guys . . ." The clerk presented the bill. Dick reached in his hip pocket, frowned, snapped his fingers, and said, "Hot damn! I forgot my wallet." Which to his partner seemed a ploy so feeble that it couldn't possibly fool [anybody]. The clerk, apparently, was not of that opinion, for he produced a blank check, and when Dick had made it out for eighty dollars more than the bill totaled, instantly paid over the difference in cash.

—Truman Capote, *In Cold Blood*

In his book *Echoes in the Darkness*,[2] Joseph Wambaugh skillfully describes a psychopathic teacher, William Bradfield, who was able to bamboozle everyone around him with his apparent erudition. *Almost* everyone, that is. Those familiar with the disciplines in which Bradfield claimed expertise were quickly able to spot his superficial knowledge of the topics. One noted that he had "a good two-line opening on any subject, but nothing more."

Of course it's not always easy to tell whether an individual is being glib or sincere, particularly when we know little about the speaker. For example, suppose a woman meets an attractive man in a bar and, while sipping a glass of wine, he says the following:

I've wasted a lot of my life. You can't get back the time. I've tried that before, to make up the time by doing more things. But things just went faster, not better. I intend to live a much more slowed-down life, and give a lot to people that I never had myself. Put some enjoyment in their lives. I don't mean thrills, I mean some substance into somebody else's life. It will probably be a woman, but it doesn't necessarily have to be a woman. Maybe a woman's kids, or maybe someone in an old folks' home. I think . . . no, I don't think . . . I *know*, it would give me a great deal of pleasure, make me feel a whole lot better about my life.

Is this individual sincere? Were the words spoken with conviction? They came from a forty-five-year-old inmate with a horrendous criminal record, a man with the highest possible score on the *Psychopathy Checklist* and who had brutalized his wife and abandoned his children.

In his book *Fatal Vision*,[3] Joe McGinniss described his relationship with Jeffrey MacDonald, a psychopathic physician convicted of killing his wife and children:

For six months following his conviction, maybe seven or eight, finding myself confronted by the most awful set of circumstances I'd ever known as a writer, and all the while being beseeched by this charming and persuasive man to believe in him, I wrestled with not only the question of his guilt but with another that was in some ways more disturbing: *if he could have done this, how could I have liked him?* [p. 668]

Jeffrey MacDonald sued McGinniss for several things, including "intentional infliction of emotional distress." Author Joseph Wambaugh testified at the trial, and said the following about MacDonald, whom he considered a psychopath:

I found him to be extremely glib . . . I had never met anyone quite as glib I don't think, and I was astonished by the manner in which [his] story was delivered. He was describing events of consummate horror, but he could describe the murders in quite graphic detail . . . in a very detached and glib and easy manner . . . I have interviewed dozens of people who were survivors of horrible crimes, some immediately after the events and some many years after, including the parents of murdered children, and I have never in all of my experience encountered someone who could describe an event like that in the almost cavalier manner that Dr. MacDonald described it. [p. 678]

Egocentric and Grandiose

"I. I. I. . . . The world continued to revolve around her as she shone—not the brightest star but the only star," said Ann Rule of Diane Downs, who in 1984 was convicted of shooting her three small children, killing one and permanently injuring the two others.[4]

Psychopaths have a narcissistic and grossly inflated view of their self-worth and importance, a truly astounding egocentricity and sense of entitlement, and see themselves as the center of the universe, as superior beings who are justified in living according to their own rules. "It's not that I don't follow the law," said one of our subjects. "I follow my own laws. I never violate my own rules." She then described these rules in terms of "looking out for number one."

When another psychopath, in prison for a variety of crimes including robbery, rape, and fraud, was asked if he had any weaknesses, he replied, "I don't have any weaknesses, except maybe I'm too caring." On a 10-point scale he rated himself "an all-round 10. I would have said 12, but that would be bragging. If I had a better education I'd be brilliant."

The grandiosity and pomposity of some psychopaths often emerges in dramatic fashion in the courtroom. For example, it is not unusual for them to criticize or fire their lawyers and to take over their own defense, usually with disastrous results."My partner got a year. I got two because of a shithead lawyer," said one of our subjects. He later handled his own appeal and saw his sentence increased to three years.

Psychopaths often come across as arrogant, shameless braggarts—self-assured, opinionated, domineering, and cocky. They love to have power and control over others and seem unable to believe that other people have valid opinions different from theirs. They appear charismatic or "electrifying" to some people.

Psychopaths are seldom embarrassed about their legal, financial, or personal problems. Rather, they see them as temporary setbacks, the results of bad luck, unfaithful friends, or an unfair and incompetent system.

Although psychopaths often claim to have specific goals, they show little understanding of the qualifications required—they have no idea how to achieve their goals and little or no chance of attaining them, given their track record and lack of sustained interest in education. The psychopathic inmate thinking about parole might outline vague plans to become a property tycoon or a lawyer for the poor. One inmate, not particularly literate, managed to copyright the title of a book he was planning to write about himself and was already counting the fortune his bestseller would bring.

Psychopaths feel that their abilities will enable them to become anything they want to be. Given the right circumstances—opportunity, luck, willing victims—their grandiosity can pay off spectacularly. For example, the psychopathic entrepreneur "thinks big," but it's usually with someone else's money.

Incarcerated for breaking and entering, one in a string of crimes dating back to early adolescence, Jack received the highest possible score on the *Psychopathy Checklist*. Typically, he began the interview with an inordinate interest in the video camera. "When do we get to see the tape? I want to see how I look, how I did." Jack then launched into a detailed lengthy account—four hours long—of his criminal history, punctuating it with constant reminders to himself that, "Oh, yeah, I've given all that up." The story that unfolded was one of constant petty thefts and con jobs—"the more people you meet the more money you can make off 'em, and they're not really victims. Hell, they always get back more than they lost in insurance anyway."

Along with the petty theft, which eventually led to burglary and armed robbery, was a history of fighting. "Oh, yeah, I've been fag-bashing since I was fourteen—but I don't do anything bad, like beating women or children. In fact, I *love* women. I think they should all stay home. I'd like all the men in the world to just die, and I'd be the only man left.

"When I get out this time, I want to have a son," Jack told our interviewer. "When he's five, I'd get the woman to completely pull out so I could raise the kid *my* way."

Asked how he had begun his career in crime, he said, "It had to do with my mother, the most beautiful person in the world. She was strong, worked hard to take care of four kids. A beautiful person. I started stealing her jewelry when I was in the fifth grade. You know, I never really knew the bitch—we went our separate ways."

Jack made a token effort to justify his life of crime—"I had to steal sometimes to get out of town, yeah, but *I'm not a fucking criminal.*" Later in the interview, however, he recalled, "I did sixteen B & Es [break and enters] in ten days. It was good, it really felt good. Felt like I was addicted and getting my fix."

"Ever tell lies?" asked the interviewer.

"Are you kidding? I lie like I breathe, one as much as the other."

Jack's interviewer, a psychologist experienced in administering the *Psychopathy Checklist,* described the interview as not only the lengthiest but most entertaining she had ever conducted. Jack was, she said, one of the most theatrical inmates she'd encountered. Although he expressed zero empathy for his victims, he clearly *loved* his crimes and seemed to be trying to impress the interviewer with his amazing feats of irresponsibility. Jack was a mile-a-minute talker, with the psychopath's characteristic ability to contradict himself from one sentence to the next. His long conviction record reflected not only his criminal versatility but his clear inability to learn from past experience.

Equally dazzling was Jack's distinct lack of realistic planning. Although he was considerably out of shape and overweight from years of prison food and cheap fast food on the outside, he told our interviewer with the confidence of a young athlete in training that he planned to become a professional swimmer when he left prison this time. He would go straight, live off his winnings, and travel on them when he retired at an early age.

Jack was thirty-eight years old at the time of the interview. Whether he had ever been a swimmer in his life was not known.

A Lack of Remorse or Guilt

Psychopaths show a stunning lack of concern for the devastating effects their actions have on others. Often they are completely forthright about the matter, calmly stating that they have no sense of guilt, are not sorry for the pain and destruction they have caused, and that there is no reason for them to be concerned.

When asked if he had any regrets about stabbing a robbery victim who subsequently spent three months in the hospital as a result of his wounds, one of our subjects replied, "Get real! He spends a few months in a hospital and I rot here. I cut him up a bit, but if I wanted to kill him I would have slit his throat. That's the kind of guy I am; I gave him a break." Asked if he regretted *any* of his crimes, he said, "I don't regret nothing. What's done is done. There must have been a reason why I did it at the time, and that is why it was done."

Before his execution, serial killer Ted Bundy spoke directly of guilt in several interviews with Stephen Michaud and Hugh Aynesworth.[5] "[Whatever] I've done in the past," he said, "you know—the emotions of omissions or commissions—*doesn't* bother me. Try to touch the past! Try to deal with the past. It's not real. It's just a dream!" [p. 284] Bundy's "dream" contained his murders of as many as a hundred young women—not only had he walked away from his past, but he extinguished the future of each of his young victims, one by one. "Guilt?" he remarked in prison. "It's this mechanism we use to control people. It's an illusion. It's a kind of social control mechanism—and it's *very* unhealthy. It does terrible things to our bodies. And there are much better ways to control our behavior than that rather extraordinary use of guilt." [p. 288]

On the other hand, psychopaths sometimes verbalize remorse but then contradict themselves in words or actions. Criminals in prison quickly learn that *remorse* is an important word. When asked if he experienced remorse over a murder he'd committed, one young inmate told us, "Yeah, sure, I feel remorse." Pressed further, he said that he didn't "feel bad inside about it."

I was once dumbfounded by the logic of an inmate who described his murder victim as having benefited from the crime by learning "a hard lesson about life."

"The guy only had himself to blame," another inmate said of the man he'd murdered in an argument about paying a bar tab. "Anybody could have seen I was in a rotten mood that night.

What did he want to go and bother me for?" He continued, "Anyway, the guy never suffered. Knife wounds to an artery are the easiest way to go."

Psychopaths' lack of remorse or guilt is associated with a remarkable ability to rationalize their behavior and to shrug off personal responsibility for actions that cause shock and disappointment to family, friends, associates, and others who have played by the rules. Usually they have handy excuses for their behavior, and in some cases they deny that it happened at all.

JACK ABBOTT GAINED prominence in the news when writer Norman Mailer helped the inmate with the publication of his book, *In the Belly of the Beast: Letters from Prison.* Abbott gained not only fame from his association with the well-known novelist and political figure; he gained his freedom as well. Shortly after his parole, Abbott got into an altercation with a waiter in a New York restaurant who had asked Abbott to leave. Abbott balked, and the two wound up behind the restaurant, where Abbott slipped a knife into the unarmed waiter, Richard Adan, wounding him fatally.

Interviewed on *A Current Affair,* a network "news magazine" television program, Abbott was asked if he felt remorse. "I don't think that's the proper word. . . . Remorse implies you did something wrong. . . . *If* I'm the one who stabbed him, it was an accident."

Abbott was convicted of the crime and sent back to prison. Some years later, Adan's wife sued him in civil court for the wrongful death of her husband, and Abbott served as his own attorney. Ricci Adan, the victim's wife, described Abbott's treatment of her on the stand: "He would say I'm sorry and then all of a sudden he would insult me."

"Everybody in that courtroom knew I was railroaded," Abbott told the TV interviewer. Regarding the depth of his conscious feelings about the death, we must draw our conclusions from these remarks: "There was no pain, it was a clean wound." Then he focused on Richard Adan himself: "He had no future as an actor—chances are he would have gone into another line of work."

The N.Y. Times News Service (June 16, 1990) reported that

> Abbott had told Ricci Adan that her husband's life was "not
> worth a dime." Nevertheless, she was awarded more than $7
> million.

Memory loss, amnesia, blackouts, multiple personality, and
temporary insanity crop up constantly in interrogations of psychopaths. For example, a well-publicized film clip from a PBS
special shows Kenneth Bianchi, one of the infamous "Hillside
Stranglers" of Los Angeles, in a pathetic and transparent pantomime of a case of multiple personality.[6]

Although sometimes a psychopath will admit to having performed the actions, he will greatly minimize or even deny the
consequences to others. An inmate with a very high score on
the *Psychopathy Checklist* said that his crimes actually had a positive effect on the victims. "The next day I'd get the newspaper
and read about a caper I'd pulled—a robbery or a rape. There'd
be interviews with the victims. They'd get their names in the
paper. Women, for example, would say nice things about me—
that I was really polite and considerate, very meticulous. I
wasn't abusive to them, you understand. Some of them thanked
me."

Another subject, up for breaking and entering for the twentieth time, said, "Sure I stole the stuff. But, hey! Those folks
were insured up the kazoo—nobody got hurt, nobody suffered.
What's the big deal? In fact, I'm doing *them* a favor by giving
them a chance to collect insurance. They'll put in for more than
that junk was worth, you know. They always do."

In an ironic twist, psychopaths frequently see *themselves* as the
real victims.

"I was made an asshole and a scapegoat . . . when I look
back I see myself more as a victim than a perpetrator." So said
John Wayne Gacy, a psychopathic serial killer who tortured and
murdered thirty-three young men and boys and buried their
bodies in the basement of his house.[7]

While discussing these murders Gacy portrayed himself as the
thirty-fourth victim. "I was the victim, I was cheated out of my
childhood." He wondered to himself if "there would be someone, somewhere who would understand how badly it had hurt
to be John Wayne Gacy."

In his book about Kenneth Taylor, the dentist who severely beat his wife on their honeymoon, cheated on her, and later battered her to death, Peter Maas quoted him as saying, "I loved her so deeply. I miss her so much. What happened was a tragedy. I lost my best lover and my best friend. . . . Why doesn't anybody understand what I've been going through?"[8]

Lack of Empathy

Many of the characteristics displayed by psychopaths—especially their egocentricity, lack of remorse, shallow emotions, and deceitfulness—are closely associated with a profound lack of empathy (an inability to construct a mental and emotional "facsimile" of another person). They seem unable to "get into the skin" or to "walk in the shoes" of others, except in a purely intellectual sense. The feelings of other people are of no concern to psychopaths.

In some respects they are like the emotionless androids depicted in science fiction, unable to imagine what real humans experience. One rapist, high on the *Psychopathy Checklist,* commented that he found it hard to empathize with his victims. "They are frightened, right? But, you see, I don't really understand it. I've been scared myself, and it wasn't unpleasant."

Psychopaths view people as little more than objects to be used for their own gratification. The weak and the vulnerable—whom they mock, rather than pity—are favorite targets. "There is no such thing, in the psychopathic universe, as the merely weak," wrote psychologist Robert Rieber. "Whoever is weak is also a sucker; that is, someone who demands to be exploited."[9]

"Oh, terrible, very unfortunate," snapped a young inmate when told of the death of a boy he had stabbed in a gang clash. "Don't try to soften me up with that crap. The little puke got what he deserved and I can't worry about it. As you can see"— he gestured toward the interrogating officers—"I've got my own problems here."

In order to survive both physically and psychologically, some normal individuals develop a degree of insensitivity to the feelings and plight of specific groups of people. For example, doctors who are too empathic toward their patients would soon become emotionally overwhelmed, and their effectiveness as physicians would be reduced. For them, insensitivity is circumscribed, confined to a specific target group. Similarly, soldiers, gang members, and terrorists may be trained—very effectively, as history has proved over and over again—to view the enemy as less-than-human, as an object without an inner life.

Psychopaths, however, display a *general* lack of empathy. They are indifferent to the rights and suffering of family members and strangers alike. If they do maintain ties with their spouses or children it is only because they see their family members as possessions, much like their stereos or automobiles. Indeed, it is difficult to avoid the conclusion that some psychopaths are more concerned with the inner workings of their cars than with the inner worlds of their "loved" ones. One of our subjects allowed her boyfriend to sexually molest her five-year-old daughter because "he wore me out. I wasn't ready for more sex that night." The woman found it difficult to understand why the authorities took her child into care. "She belongs to me. Her welfare is my business." She didn't protest very much, however—certainly not as much as she did when her car was impounded, during the custody hearing, for nonpayment of traffic tickets.

Because of their inability to appreciate the feelings of others, some psychopaths are capable of behavior that normal people find not only horrific but baffling. For example, they can torture and mutilate their victims with about the same sense of concern that we feel when we carve a turkey for Thanksgiving dinner.

However, except in movies and books, very few psychopaths commit crimes of this sort. Their callousness typically emerges in less dramatic, though still devastating, ways: parasitically bleeding other people of their possessions, savings, and dignity; aggressively doing and taking what they want; shamefully neglecting the physical and emotional welfare of their families; engaging in an unending series of casual, impersonal, and trivial sexual relationships; and so forth.

CONNIE IS FIFTEEN, hovering between childhood and womanhood, sometimes darting from one to another in a single day. She is a virgin but attuned to her burgeoning sexuality like one listening intently to a song inside her head. But on a hot sultry day when her family has left her to herself, a stranger comes to her house—a stranger who says he's been watching her.

"I'm your lover, honey," [he tells her]. "You don't know what that is but you will. . . . I know all about you. . . . I'll tell you how it is, I'm always nice at first, the first time. I'll hold you so tight you won't think you have to try to get away or pretend anything because you'll know you can't. And I'll come inside you where it's all secret and you'll give in to me and you'll love me—" . . . "I'm going to call the police—". . . . [Out] of his mouth came a fast spat curse, an aside not meant for her to hear. But even this "Christ!" sounded forced. Then he began to smile again. She watched his smile come, awkward as if he were smiling from inside a mask. His whole face was a mask, she thought wildly, tanned down to his throat. "This is how it is, honey: you come out and we'll drive away, have a nice ride. But if you don't come out we're gonna wait till your people come home and then they're all going to get it. . . . "My sweet little blue-eyed girl," he said in a half-sung sigh that had nothing to do with her brown eyes. . . . [Joyce Carol Oates, "Where Are You Going, Where Have You Been?"]

Deceitful and Manipulative

Lying, deceiving, and manipulation are natural talents for psychopaths.

With their powers of imagination in gear and focused on themselves, psychopaths appear amazingly unfazed by the possibility—or even by the certainty—of being found out. When caught in a lie or challenged with the truth, they are seldom perplexed or embarrassed—they simply change their stories or attempt to rework the facts so that they appear to be consistent with the lie. The results are a series of contradictory statements and a thoroughly confused listener. Much of the lying seems to have no motivation other than what psychologist Paul Ekman refers to as a "duping delight."[10]

"I'M A VERY feeling person. You can't help but fall in love with these kids," said Genene Jones, convicted of murdering two infants and suspected of killing more than a dozen others. A San Antonio practical nurse, she administered life-threatening drugs to neonates in an intensive care unit in order to put herself in the role of hero by bringing them back from the "brink of death." Her "bewitching presence," air of supreme confidence, and convincing demeanor, along with a shocking medical cover-up, allowed her to ply her trade in spite of widespread suspicions about her role in many infant deaths and near-fatal emergencies. In conversation with author Peter Elkind, Jones complained that she was "being made a scapegoat because [I] was so abrasive. 'My mouth got me into this,' Genene said with a grin. 'And my mouth's going to get me out of it.'" Like all psychopaths, she showed a remarkable ability to manipulate the truth to suit her own purposes. "By the end of our conversation," wrote Elkind, "Genene had completed an account of her life that was astonishingly different from what I had gathered from dozens of those who had known her. It clashed with reality not merely on the basis of her guilt ... but on a thousand details, small and unimportant, except as they loomed in Genene's image of herself. Genene was contradicting not only during recollections of others and a voluminous written record, but facts she had told me *herself* four years earlier. . . . For her, the lines between truth and fiction, between good and evil, between right and wrong, did not matter." [Peter Elkind, *The Death Shift*]

Psychopaths seem proud of their ability to lie. When asked if she lied easily, one woman with a high score on the *Psychopathy Checklist* laughed and replied, "I'm the best. I'm really good at it, I think because I sometimes admit to something bad about myself. They'd think, well, if she's admitting to that she must be telling the truth about the rest." She also said that she sometimes "salts the mine" with a nugget of truth. "If they think some of what you say is true, they usually think it's all true."

Many observers get the impression that psychopaths sometimes are unaware that they're lying; it is as if the words take on a life of their own, unfettered by the speaker's knowledge that the observer is aware of the facts. The psychopath's indifference to being identified as a liar is truly extraordinary; it causes the listener to wonder about the speaker's sanity. More often, though, the listener is taken in.

At the workshops we conduct for mental health and forensic workers, the members of the audience often express surprise when they learn the conviction history of the subject in one of our videotaped interviews. The subject is a good-looking, fast-talking twenty-four-year-old man with a million post release plans and a seemingly inexhaustible supply of untapped talents. In rapid succession he convincingly described having done the following:

- left home at age eight

- started flying at age eleven; pilot's license at age fifteen

- was a commercial pilot with twin-engine and full instrumentation experience

- lived in nine different countries in four continents

- managed an apartment building

- had his own roofing company

- ran a ranch for a year

- worked as a forest-fire fighter for six months

- spent two years in the coast guard

- was a captain on an eighty-foot charter boat

- was a deep-sea diver for four months

Presently serving time for murder, he has been denied parole four times but still has lots of plans: to get into property development, to sell time-share vacation condos, to get a commercial pilot's license, and so on. He also plans to live with his parents, whom he hasn't seen in seventeen years. Referring to psychological tests he had taken, he said, "I IQ'd out, passed all the tests with flying colors. They rated me as superior intelligence."

For obvious reasons, we've nicknamed him "motor-mouth."

His philosophy? "If you throw enough shit, some of it will stick." It seems to work, because he leaves even sophisticated observers convinced of his sincerity. For example, one interviewer's notes contained statements such as: "very impressive"; "sincere and forthright"; possesses good interpersonal skills"; "intelligent and articulate." What the interviewer learned after reading his files, however, was that virtually none of what the inmate had told him was true. Needless to say, this man's score on the *Psychopathy Checklist* was very high.

Given their glibness and the facility with which they lie, it is not surprising that psychopaths successfully cheat, bilk, defraud, con, and manipulate people and have not the slightest compunction about doing so. They are often forthright in describing themselves as con men, hustlers, or fraud artists. Their statements often reveal their belief that the world is made up of "givers and takers," predators and prey, and that it would be very foolish not to exploit the weaknesses of others. In addition, they can be very astute at determining what those weaknesses are and at using them for their own benefit. "I like to con people. I'm conning you now," said one of our subjects, a forty-five-year-old man serving his first prison sentence for stock fraud.

Some of their operations are elaborate and well thought out, whereas others are quite simple: stringing along several women at the same time, or convincing family members and friends that money is needed "to bail me out of a jam." Whatever the scheme, it is carried off in a cool, self-assured, brazen manner.

"Oh, the seventies," reminisced a social activist interviewed for this book. "I ran a halfway house for ex-cons, and split my time between counseling these guys, finding them jobs, and raising money to keep the thing going. One guy acted like my best friend—I really liked him; he could come on like a pussycat. And then he just up and cleaned us out. Not once but twice he completely emptied the place: typewriters, furniture, food, office supplies, everything. After the first time, he somehow managed to convince me he was ashamed and sorry, and I can't believe I fell for that remorse bit, but I did. About a month later he forged a check and all but closed out our bank account. This time he disappeared, and that was the end of *that* venture. There I was standing in the bank clutching a bunch of overdraft notices and talking fast. It still galls me, because I was no easy touch. I was used to being around some pretty tough guys, and I thought I knew my way around the block with the likes of them. I never realized I could be conned so thoroughly, but there I was in a few weeks looking for a job for myself."

The capacity to con friend and foe alike makes it a simple matter for psychopaths to perpetrate fraud, embezzlement, and impersonation, to promote phony stocks and worthless property, and to carry out swindles of all sorts, large and small. One of our subjects told of strolling along a dock when he spied a young couple looking at a large sailboat with a For Sale sign on it. He walked over to the couple, smoothly introduced himself as the boat's owner—"a complete load of baloney," he told us—and invited them aboard to look around. After an enjoyable hour on the boat, the couple made an offer to buy. Once the terms had been negotiated, he agreed to meet the couple at the bank the next day and asked for a $1,500 deposit to seal the deal. After a friendly parting, he cashed their deposit check and never saw them again.

"Money grows on trees," said another psychopath, a woman with a long history of frauds and petty thefts. "They say it doesn't but it does. I don't *want* to do it to people, it's just so *easy!*"

In the same vein, psychopaths in prison often learn to use the correctional facilities to their own advantage and to help shape a positive image of themselves for the benefit of the parole board. They take classes and degree courses, enroll in programs for drug and alcohol abuse, join religious and quasi-religious groups, and adopt whatever self-improvement fad is in favor— not to "rehabilitate" themselves but to *look* as if they are doing so. It's not unusual, for example, for a particularly adept manipulator to declare himself "born again" in the Christian sense— not only to convince the parole board of his sincere resolve to reform but to exploit the elaborate and well-meaning born-again community for its support . . . not to mention its material resources. And now that "cycle of abuse" theories have become widely accepted, many psychopaths are eager to attribute their faults and problems to childhood abuse. Although their claims may be difficult to verify, there is never a shortage of well-meaning people ready to take them at face value.

CONSIDER: HOW DO you get people to do what you want them to do? Now add an element: How do you do that when what you want them to do goes against every inclination in their own personalities and everything they grew up knowing was wrong, dangerous, unthinkable—for example, getting into a car with a man you've never seen before, especially if you're a young, pretty woman far from home?

Ted Bundy, perhaps the most visible and widely known serial killer the United States has ever produced—executed in 1989 for the last in a long string of brutal murders of young women—must have pondered that question long and hard from every angle. He must have drawn on all his powers of observation, which were considerable and were sharpened by his study of psychology in college. He must have plumbed the depths of his knowledge and experience of people's problems and vulnerabilities—these were honed by the time he spent as a peer counselor on a crisis hotline. We can't know for sure what went on in Ted Bundy's mind when he began to lure his victims into his car and drive them to the site of their murders. But we can assume that the above suppositions are true based on the solutions he came up with—variations on a theme that he reportedly tried over and over again, to get it right.

Ted Bundy bought himself a pair of crutches and even went so far as to give the appearance of putting his leg in a cast. Thus temporarily "disabled," he asked for assistance from sympathetic young women who might cross the street to avoid a pass but who apparently readily stopped to lend a hand to a man with a broken leg. Bundy varied the theme—sometimes his arm was in a sling and he found his willing victim on a busy street; sometimes, with his leg the problem, he targeted young women at recreational areas and gained their aid in securing his boat—"It's just down the road"—to his car. In a terrible way, the ploy was a stroke of genius. Occasionally it failed and the woman he stopped refused to follow him, but, as recounted in Ann Rule's book *The Stranger Beside Me*, it worked very often indeed.

Rule's book is a study of Bundy's highly refined skill at using his good looks and smooth charm to win the trust of women. In an amazing coincidence, Rule and Bundy worked the same shift on a crisis line for several years before she was called in to write up cases for the police department on a then-unidentified serial killer of young women. As the body count mounted, Rule's suspicions began to rise. But to surface, they had to worm their way through her memories of Bundy's sympathetic and—as her prose makes clear—sexually attractive presence at the desk across from hers on the night shift. That Rule left her work as a police writer to become a bestselling crime writer turned this peculiar coincidence into an opportunity for her to show Bundy's power over others from the inside. The result? A strange and eerie book about a psychopath who said, in answer to a television interviewer who asked whether Bundy thought he deserved to die, "Good question. I think society deserves to be protected from me and from people like me."

Shallow Emotions

"I'm the most cold-blooded son of a bitch that you'll ever meet."[11] So Ted Bundy described himself to the police following his final arrest.

Psychopaths seem to suffer a kind of emotional poverty that limits the range and depth of their feelings. While at times they appear cold and unemotional, they are prone to dramatic, shallow, and short-lived displays of feeling. Careful observers are left with the impression that they are play-acting and that little is going on below the surface.

Sometimes they claim to experience strong emotions but are unable to describe the subtleties of various affective states. For example, they equate love with sexual arousal, sadness with frustration, and anger with irritability. "I believe in emotions: hate, anger, lust, and greed," said Richard Ramirez, the "Night Stalker."[12]

Remarks like the following from Diane Downs, who shot her three small children, should cause people to ponder their sheer inappropriateness and to wonder at the quality of the underlying feelings. Years after her conviction, Downs still insists that her children, and she herself, were actually shot by a "bushy-haired stranger." About surviving the shooting herself (she sustained an injury to her arm, which the jury concluded was self-inflicted), Downs responded:

> Everybody says, "You sure are lucky!" Well, I don't feel very lucky. I couldn't tie my damned shoes for about two months! It is very painful, it is still painful, I have a steel plate in my arm—I will for a year and a half. The scar is going to be there forever. I'm going to remember that night for the rest of my life whether I want to or not. I don't think I was very lucky. I think my kids were lucky. If I had been shot the way they were, we all would have died.[13]

The apparent lack of normal affect and emotional depth led psychologists J. H. Johns and H. C. Quay to say that the psychopath "knows the words but not the music."[14] For example, in a rambling book about hate, violence, and rationalizations for his behavior, Jack Abbott made this revealing comment: "There are emotions—a whole spectrum of them—that I know only through words, through reading and in my immature imagination. I can *imagine* I feel these emotions (know, therefore, what they are), but *I do not*. At age thirty-seven I am barely a precocious child. My passions are those of a boy."[15]

Many clinicians have commented that the emotions of psychopaths are so shallow as to be little more than *proto-emotions*: primitive responses to immediate needs. (I'll discuss the most recent research findings on this topic in later chapters.) For example, one of our psychopathic subjects, a twenty-eight-year-old "enforcer" for a loan shark, had this to say about his job: "Say I have to heavy someone who won't pay up. First I make myself angry." When asked if this anger was different from the way he feels when someone insults him or tries to take advantage of him, he replied, "No. It's all the same. It's programmed, all worked out. I could get angry right now. It's easy to turn on and off."

Another psychopath in our research said that he did not really understand what others meant by "fear." However, "When I rob a bank," he said, "I notice that the teller shakes or becomes tongue-tied. One barfed all over the money. She must have been pretty messed up inside, but I don't know why. If someone pointed a gun at me I guess I'd be afraid, but I wouldn't throw up." When asked to describe how he *would* feel in such a situation, his reply contained no reference to bodily sensations. He said things such as, "I'd give you the money"; "I'd think of ways to get the drop on you"; "I'd try and get my ass out of there." When asked how he would *feel*, not what he would think or do, he seemed perplexed. Asked if he ever felt his heart pound or his stomach churn, he replied, "Of course! I'm not a robot. I really get pumped up when I have sex or when I get into a fight."

Laboratory experiments using biomedical recorders have shown that psychopaths lack the physiological responses normally associated with fear.[16] The significance of this finding is that, for most people, the fear produced by threats of pain or punishment is an unpleasant emotion and a powerful motivator of behavior. Fear keeps us from doing some things—"Do it *and* you'll be sorry"—but it also makes us do other things—"Do it *or* you'll be sorry." In each case, it is emotional awareness of the consequences that impels us to take a particular course of action. Not so with psychopaths; they merrily plunge on, perhaps knowing what might happen but not really caring.

"HIS SOCIAL STATUS notwithstanding, he is truly one of the most dangerous sociopaths I have ever seen," said the Superior Court Judge after sentencing respected 37-year-old San Jose attorney Norman Russell Sjonborg for the brutal slaying of one of his clients from whom he had embezzled money. His third wife, Terry, who initially had provided him with an alibi for the crime, said that when she first met him, "He seemed like a nice guy, soft-spoken and exceedingly charming." But she also noted, "From the start Russell spoke about this emotional void, an inability to feel things like everyone else; to know when to cry, when to feel joy." Terry also commented that he "led a kind of paint-by-numbers emotional life," and that "he read self-help psychology books to learn the appropriate emotional responses to everyday events."

As their marriage began to break down Russell tried to convince his wife that she was going mad. "I would go into [counseling] sessions a basket case," she said, "and Russell would sit there calm and gracious and rational, and he'd turn to the therapist and say, 'See what I have to put up with?' and I'd shout and scream and say, 'It's not me. He's the crazy one!' But the counselor bought Russell's act and said we could never make progress as a couple if I blamed everything on my husband."

Later Russell worked out several scenarios for handling his problems with his wife and wrote them down on a piece of paper: "Do nothing"; "File for Paternity/Conciliation Court"; "Take girls w/o killing"; "Take girls Killing 4"; "Kill Girls and Justin." His probation officer commented that the list revealed "the mind of a man who could contemplate killing his own children with the detachment of someone considering various auto-insurance policies. It is the laundry list of a man without a soul."

Referring to Russell's murder of Phyllis Wilde, his wife said, "I saw him just hours after he had bludgeoned [her] to death. There was nothing in his behavior to betray him. . . . No fear, no remorse, nothing."

In a statement to the Judge, Terry pleaded, "Please see the animal inside him; do not see the socially acceptable persona that he creates on the outside." She expressed her fear that he would eventually track her down. "I know what will happen. He'll be a model prisoner, endear himself to the other prisoners and the people in charge. Eventually he'll be transferred to a minimum-security facility. And then he'll escape." [From an article by Rider McDowell in the January 26, 1992, edition of *Image*]

For most of us, fear and apprehension are associated with a variety of unpleasant bodily sensations, such as sweating of the hands, a "pounding" heart, dry mouth, muscle tenseness or weakness, trembles, and "butterflies" in the stomach. Indeed, we often describe fear in terms of the bodily sensations that accompany them: "I was so terrified my heart leapt into my throat"; "I tried to speak but my mouth went dry"; and so forth.

These bodily sensations do not form part of what psychopaths experience as fear. For them, fear—like most other emotions—is incomplete, shallow, largely cognitive in nature, and without the physiological turmoil or "coloring" that most of us find distinctly unpleasant and wish to avoid or reduce.

Chapter 4

The Profile: Lifestyle

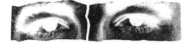

> The total pattern of the psychopath's personality differentiates him from the normal criminal. His aggression is more intense, his impulsivity more pronounced, his emotional reactions more shallow. His guiltlessness, however, is the critical distinguishing trait. The normal criminal has an internalized, albeit warped, set of values. If he violates these standards he feels guilt.
> —McCord and McCord. *The Psychopath: An Essay on the Criminal Mind*[1]

In chapter 3 I described the way psychopaths think and feel about themselves and others—the emotional/interpersonal symptoms noted in my *Psychopathy Checklist*. But this is only one facet of the syndrome. The other facet, described in this chapter, and comprised of the remaining symptoms in the *Psychopathy Checklist*, is a chronically unstable and aimless lifestyle marked by casual and flagrant violations of social norms and expectations. Together, these two facets—one depicting feelings and relationships, the other social deviance—provide a comprehensive picture of the psychopathic personality.

Impulsive

Psychopaths are unlikely to spend much time weighing the pros and cons of a course of action or considering the possible consequences. "I did it because I felt like it," is a common response.

Texas murderer Gary Gilmore gained national attention for legally pursuing his own execution—and for succeeding: In 1977 he was the first person executed in the United States in ten years. In response to the question, "If you hadn't been caught that night, do you think there would have been a third or fourth murder?" Gilmore answered, "Until I got caught or shot to death by the police or something like that . . . *I wasn't thinkin', I wasn't plannin', I was just doin'.* It was a damned shame for those two guys. . . . I'm just saying that murder vents rage. Rage is not reason. The murders were without reason. Don't try to understand murder by using reason." [italics mine][2]

More than displays of temper, impulsive acts often result from an aim that plays a central role in most of the psychopath's behavior: to achieve immediate satisfaction, pleasure, or relief. "The psychopath is like an infant, absorbed in his own needs, vehemently demanding satiation," wrote psychologists William and Joan McCord.[3] At an early age most children have already begun to postpone pleasure, compromising with restrictions in the environment. A parent can generally use a promise to put off satisfying a two-year-old's desires, at least temporarily, but psychopaths never seem to learn this lesson—they do not modify their desires; they ignore the needs of others.

So, family members, employers, and co-workers typically find themselves standing around asking themselves what happened—jobs are quit, relationships broken off, plans changed, houses ransacked, people hurt, often for what appears little more than a whim. As the husband of a psychopath I studied put it: "She got up and left the table, and that was the last I saw of her for two months."

One of our subjects, who scored high on the *Psychopathy Checklist*, said that while walking to a party he decided to buy a case of beer, but realized that he had left his wallet at home six or seven blocks away. Not wanting to walk back, he picked up a heavy piece of wood and robbed the nearest gas station, seriously injuring the attendant.

Psychopaths tend to live day-to-day and to change their plans frequently. They give little serious thought to the future and worry about it even less. Nor do they generally show much concern about how little they have done with their lives. "Look, I'm a drifter, a nomad—I hate being pinned down," is a typical remark.

One man we interviewed used an analogy to explain why he "lived for the moment." "We're always being told to drive defensively, to mentally plan escape routes in case of an emergency, to look well ahead of the car just in front of us. But hey, it's the car just in front of us that's the real danger, and if we always look too far ahead we'll hit it. If I always think about tomorrow I won't be able to live today."

Poor Behavior Controls

Besides being impulsive—doing things on the spur of the moment—psychopaths are highly reactive to perceived insults or slights. Most of us have powerful inhibitory controls over our behavior; even if we would like to respond aggressively we are usually able to "keep the lid on." In psychopaths, these inhibitory controls are weak, and the slightest provocation is sufficient to overcome them. As a result, psychopaths are short-tempered or hot-headed and tend to respond to frustration, failure, discipline, and criticism with sudden violence, threats, and verbal abuse. They take offense easily and become angry and aggressive over trivialities, and often in a context that appears inappropriate to others. But their outbursts, extreme as they may be, are generally short-lived, and they quickly resume acting as if nothing out of the ordinary has happened.

Carl, an inmate, made a call to his wife from the prison pay phone and learned that she wouldn't be able to visit him that weekend and bring him the cigarettes and food he'd requested because she hadn't been able to find anyone to watch their children. "You fucking bitch," he yelled into the phone. "I'll kill you, you whore." He added a convincing touch to the threat by punching the wall and bloodying his knuckles. Immediately after hanging up, though, he began to laugh and joke with some of his fellow inmates, and seemed genuinely perplexed when a guard, who had heard part of the telephone conversation, charged him with verbal abuse and threatening behavior.

An inmate in line for dinner was accidentally bumped by another inmate, whom he proceeded to beat senseless. The attacker then stepped back into his place in line as if nothing had happened. Despite the fact that he faced solitary confinement as punishment for the infraction, his only comment when asked to explain himself was, "I was pissed off. He stepped into my space. I did what I had to do."

In a classic case of "displacement," one of our subjects had an argument with a very large bouncer at a local pub, lost his temper, and punched a bystander. The victim fell backward, struck his head on the edge of a table, and died two days later. "I saw red and this guy was laughing at me." He blamed the victim for making him mad and accused the hospital of negligence for letting the victim die.

Although psychopaths have a "hair trigger" and readily initiate aggressive displays, their ensuing behavior is not out of control. On the contrary, when psychopaths "blow their stack" it is as if they are having a temper tantrum; they know exactly what they are doing. Their aggressive displays are "cold"; they lack the intense emotional arousal experienced by others when they lose their temper. For example, when asked if he ever lost control when he got mad, an inmate who scored high on the *Psychopathy Checklist* replied, "No. I keep myself in control. Like, I decide how much I want to hurt the guy."

It's not unusual for psychopaths to inflict serious physical or emotional damage on others, sometimes routinely, and yet refuse to acknowledge that they have a problem controlling their tempers. In most cases, they see their aggressive displays as natural responses to provocation.

Need for Excitement

Psychopaths have an ongoing and excessive need for excitement—they long to live in the fast lane or "on the edge," where the action is. In many cases the action involves breaking the rules.

In *The Mask of Sanity* (p. 208) Hervey Cleckley describes a psychopathic psychiatrist who never broke the law to any significant extent, but who was unable to tolerate the self-containment required by professional life and went on periodic binges. During these weekend outbursts he would shatter his image as a professional care giver by degrading, insulting, and even physically threatening any woman who found herself in his company.

Some psychopaths use a wide variety of drugs as part of their general search for something new and exciting, and they often move from place to place and job to job searching for a fresh buzz. One adolescent we interviewed had a novel way of keeping his juices flowing: Somehow, weekend after weekend, he persuaded his buddies to play "chicken" with a freight train on a bridge over a river. The group would stand on the bridge facing the train, and the first to jump would have to buy beer for the rest. Our subject, a highly persuasive, machine-gun conversationalist, never once had to buy the beer.

Many psychopaths describe "doing crime" for excitement or thrills. When asked if she ever did crazy or dangerous things just for fun, one of our female subjects replied, "Yeah, lots of things. But what I find most exciting is walking through airports with drugs. Christ! What a high!"

A male psychopath said he enjoyed his job as an "enforcer" for a drug dealer because of "the adrenaline rush. When I'm not on the job I'll go into a bar and walk up to someone and blow smoke in his face, and we'll go outside and fight, and usually he ends up liking me and we'll go back in and have a drink or something."

The television documentary *Diabolical Minds* contained an interesting segment on G. Daniel Walker, a criminal with a long record of fraud, robbery, rape, and murder, and a penchant for bringing lawsuits against everyone in sight.[4] Interviewed by former FBI agent Robert Ressler, Walker offered this comment: "There is a certain excitement when you have escaped from a major penitentiary and you know the red lights are behind you and you know the sirens are going. There is a certain excitement that you just . . . it's better than sex. Oh, it's exciting."

The flip side of this yearning for excitement is an inability to tolerate routine or monotony. Psychopaths are easily bored. You are not likely to find them engaged in occupations or activities that are dull, repetitive, or that require intense concentration over long periods. I can imagine that psychopaths might function reasonably well as air-traffic controllers, but only while things are hectic and fast paced. During slow periods they would likely goof off or go to sleep, assuming that they even showed up for work.

ARE PSYCHOPATHS PARTICULARLY well suited for dangerous professions? David Cox, a former student of mine and now a psychology professor at Simon Fraser University, doesn't think so. He studied British bomb-disposal experts in Northern Ireland, beginning the research with the expectation that because psychopaths are "cool under fire" and have a strong need for excitement they would excel at the job. But he found that the soldiers who performed the exacting and dangerous task of defusing or dismantling IRA bombs referred to psychopaths as "cowboys," unreliable and impulsive individuals who lacked the perfectionism and attention to detail needed to stay alive on the job. Most were filtered out during training, and those who slipped through didn't last long.

It is just as unlikely that psychopaths would make good spies, terrorists, or mobsters, simply because their impulsiveness, concern only for the moment, and lack of allegiance to people or causes make them unpredictable, careless, and undependable—likely to be "loose cannons."

Lack of Responsibility

Obligations and commitments mean nothing to psychopaths. Their good intentions—"I'll never cheat on you again"—are promises written on the wind.

Truly horrendous credit histories, for example, reveal the

lightly taken debt, the shrugged-off loan, the empty pledge to contribute to a child's support. "That little girl means everything to me. . . . I'd do *anything* to see that she has everything I never had in my childhood." A social worker and ex-wife would receive such remarks with justifiable skepticism when their efforts to collect court-ordered child support from the psychopath have failed from day 1.

The irresponsibility and unreliability of psychopaths extend to every part of their lives. Their performance on the job is erratic, with frequent absences, misuse of company resources, violations of company policy, and general untrustworthiness. They do not honor formal or implied commitments to people, organizations, or principles.

In her book on Diane Downs, Ann Rule described a pattern of irresponsible parental behavior that is typical of psychopaths.[5] Downs would often leave her young children alone when there was no babysitter available. The children, ranging in age from fifteen months to six years, were described by neighbors as hungry, emotionally starved, and generally neglected (they were seen playing outside in winter without shoes or coats). Downs professed to love her children, but her callous indifference to their physical and emotional welfare argues otherwise.

This indifference to the welfare of children—their own as well as those of the man or woman they happen to be living with at the time—is a common theme in our files of psychopaths. Psychopaths see children as an inconvenience. Some, like Diane Downs, insist that they care a great deal for their children, but their actions belie their words. Typically, they leave children on their own for extended periods or in the care of unreliable sitters. One of our subjects and her husband left their one-month-old infant with an alcoholic friend. The friend became drunk and passed out. When he awoke he forgot that he was babysitting and left. The parents returned some eight hours later to find that their child had been apprehended by the authorities. The mother was outraged by this violation of her parental rights and accused the authorities of depriving the child of her love and affection—a position she maintained even after she was told that the baby was severely malnourished.

Psychopaths do not hesitate to use the resources of family

and friends to bail them out of difficulty. One of our subjects, a woman with a long history of disappointing her parents, induced them to put up their house for her bail following a charge of drug trafficking. She skipped bail, and her parents are now fighting to keep their home.

Psychopaths are not deterred by the possibility that their actions may cause hardship or risk for others. A twenty-five-year-old inmate in one of our studies has received more than twenty convictions for dangerous driving, driving while impaired, leaving the scene of an accident, driving without a license, and criminal negligence causing death. When asked if he would continue to drive following his release from prison, he replied, "Why not? Sure I drive fast, but I'm good at it. It takes two to have an accident."

A physician in a western state recently called to inquire about using the *Psychopathy Checklist* in a study of patients who tested positive for the HIV virus, a precursor of AIDS. In his experience some patients with the HIV virus continued to have unprotected sex with healthy, unsuspecting partners. He wanted to evaluate his clinical impression that many of these people were psychopaths who cared little about the horrendous implications of their irresponsible behavior.

An industrial psychologist commented to me that nuclear power plants carefully screen prospective employees, for obvious reasons. However, he volunteered, the usual screening procedures—interviews, personality tests, letters of reference—do not always succeed in detecting a class of individuals notorious for their unreliability and irresponsibility—namely, psychopaths.

Psychopaths are frequently successful in talking their way out of trouble—"I've learned my lesson"; "You have my word that it won't happen again"; "It was simply a big misunderstanding"; "Trust me." They are almost as successful in convincing the criminal justice system of their good intentions and their trustworthiness. Although they frequently manage to obtain probation, a suspended sentence, or early release from prison, they simply ignore the conditions imposed by the courts. That is, even when directly under the yoke of the criminal justice system, they do not meet their obligations.

PSYCHOPATHS USUALLY DON'T get along well with one another. The last thing an egocentric, selfish, demanding, callous person wants is someone just like him. Two stars is one too many. Occasionally, however, psychopaths become temporary partners in crime—a grim symbiosis with unfortunate consequences for other people. Generally, one member of the pair is a "talker" who gets his or her way through charm, deceit, and manipulation, whereas the other is a "doer" who prefers direct action—intimidation and force. As long as their interests are complementary, they make a formidable pair.

Some examples from my files illustrate the point. In one case, two young male psychopaths were introduced at a party. One—the talker—was trying to con a minor drug dealer into letting him have some cocaine on credit, without success. The other—the doer—overheard the conversation and, as he put it, "grabbed the pusher by the balls and convinced him to provide a free sample for me and my friend." Thus began a year-long drug-dealing partnership. The talker made the contacts and arranged the deals; the doer broke legs. When the talker was caught, he immediately made a deal with the prosecutor and turned his partner in.

In another case, a young woman, a smooth-talking, parasitic psychopath, constantly complained to her friends that her parents were not contributing enough to her already lavish lifestyle. She met a middle-aged man, an aggressive, hostile psychopath, who said, "Why not do something about it?" Together, they hatched a plot in which the man would break into the woman's house and kill her parents. The woman, meanwhile, would be out of town with friends. The plot fell apart when the woman bragged to her friends that she would soon be rich. Word got to the police, who tapped the woman's telephone line and gathered enough evidence to charge the pair with conspiracy to commit murder. Each tried to plea-bargain by testifying against the other.

Sometimes a psychopath and a borderline psychotic join in a bizarre but deadly partnership, with the former using the latter as a killing tool. A well-known example was provided in Truman Capote's account of Richard Hickock and Perry Smith, executed for murdering four members of the Clutter family in 1959

(*In Cold Blood*). Hickock had all the markings of a smooth-talking psychopath, whereas Smith was diagnosed as "nearly . . . a paranoid schizophrenic." As reported by Capote, Hickock viewed Smith as a natural killer and reasoned that "such a gift could, under his supervision, be profitably exploited" [p. 69]. True to form, Hickock put the blame for the murders on his partner: "It was Perry. I couldn't stop him. He killed them all." [p. 260]

Early Behavior Problems

Most psychopaths begin to exhibit serious behavioral problems at an early age. These might include persistent lying, cheating, theft, fire setting, truancy, class disruption, substance abuse, vandalism, violence, bullying, running away, and precocious sexuality. Because many children exhibit some of these behaviors at one time or another, especially children raised in violent neighborhoods or in disrupted or abusive families, it is important to emphasize that the psychopath's history of such behaviors is more extensive and serious than that of most others, even when compared with those of siblings and friends raised in similar settings. An example of the psychopathic child is one who comes from an otherwise well-adjusted family and starts to steal, take drugs, cut school, and have sexual experiences by age ten or twelve.

Early cruelty to animals is usually a sign of serious emotional or behavioral problems. Milwaukee serial killer Jeffrey Dahmer, for example, stunned classmates and neighbors by leaving a trail of grim clues to his preoccupations: the head of a dog impaled on a stick, frogs and cats staked to trees, and a group of animal skeletons kept as a collection.[6]

Adult psychopaths usually describe their childhood cruelty to animals as ordinary events, matter-of-fact, even enjoyable. A man who scored high on the *Psychopathy Checklist* chuckled as he told us that when he was ten or eleven he shot "an irritating mutt" with a pellet gun. "I shot him in the ass and he cried and crawled around awhile and died."

Another subject, serving time for fraud, told us that as a child he would put a noose around the neck of a cat, tie the other end of the string to the top of a pole, and bat the cat around the pole with a tennis racket. He said that his sister raised puppies and he would kill the ones she didn't want to keep. "I'd tie them to a rail and use their heads for baseball practice," he said, smiling slightly.

Cruelty to other children—including siblings—is often part of the young psychopath's inability to experience the sort of empathy that checks normal people's impulses to inflict pain, even when enraged. "The shocking things he did to his baby sister's doll felt like warnings, but we brushed them aside," one mother told me. "But when he actually tried to smother his sister in her crib and snipped the skin of her neck with a pair of scissors, we realized with horror that we should have trusted our worst intuitions from the start."

Although not all adult psychopaths exhibited this degree of cruelty in their youth, virtually all routinely got themselves into a wide range of difficulties: lying, theft, vandalism, promiscuity, and so forth.

Interestingly, however, the media frequently report that witnesses and neighbors are taken completely by surprise in reaction to some senseless crime: "I just can't believe he was capable of doing a thing like that—there was absolutely no hint that he would do it." Reactions of this sort reflect not only psychopaths' power to manipulate others' impressions of themselves but the witnesses' ignorance of their early history.

Adult Antisocial Behavior

Psychopaths consider the rules and expectations of society inconvenient and unreasonable, impediments to the behavioral expression of their inclinations and wishes. They make their own rules, both as children and as adults. Impulsive, deceitful children who lack empathy and see the world as their oyster will be much the same as adults. The lifelong continuity of the self-serving, antisocial behavior of psychopaths is truly amazing.

To a large extent, this continuity is responsible for the findings, by many researchers, that the early appearance of antisocial actions is a good predictor of adult behavioral problems and criminality.[7]

Many of the antisocial acts of psychopaths lead to criminal convictions. Even within prison populations psychopaths stand out, largely because their antisocial and illegal activities are *more varied and frequent* than are those of other criminals. Psychopaths tend to have no particular affinity, or "specialty," for any one type of crime but tend to try everything. This criminal versatility is well illustrated in the television program, described earlier in this chapter, in which Robert Ressler interviewed G. Daniel Walker.[8] Following is a brief exchange from that interview:

"How long is your rap sheet?"

"I would think the current one would probably be about twenty-nine or thirty pages."

"Twenty-nine or thirty pages! Charles Manson's is only five."

"But he was only a killer."

What Walker meant was that he himself was not only a killer but a criminal of enormous versatility, a fact of which he seemed very proud. He openly boasted of having committed more than three hundred crimes in which he had not been caught.

Not all psychopaths end up in jail. Many of the things they do escape detection or prosecution, or are on the "shady side of the law." For them, antisocial behavior may consist of phony stock promotions, questionable business and professional practices, spouse or child abuse, and so forth. Many others do things that, although not illegal, are unethical, immoral, or harmful to others: philandering, cheating on a spouse, financial or emotional neglect of family members, irresponsible use of company resources or funds, to name but a few. The problem with behaviors of this sort is that they are difficult to document and evaluate without the active cooperation of family, friends, acquaintances, and business associates.

The Complete Picture

Of course, psychopaths are not the only ones who lead so-cially deviant lifestyles. For example, many criminals have some of the characteristics described in this chapter, but because they are capable of feeling guilt, remorse, empathy, and strong emo-tions, they are not considered psychopaths. A diagnosis of psy-chopathy is made *only* when there is solid evidence that the individual matches the complete profile—that is, has most of the symptoms described in *both* this chapter and the preceding one.

Recently, an ex-con offered me his opinion of the *Psychop-athy Checklist:* he wasn't too impressed! Now middle-aged, he had spent much of his early adult life in prison, where he was once diagnosed as a psychopath. Here are his responses:

- *Glib and superficial*—"What is negative about articulation skills?"
- *Egocentric and grandiose*—"How can I attain something if I don't reach high?"
- *Lack of empathy*—"Empathy toward an enemy is a sign of weakness."
- *Deceitful and manipulative*—"Why be truthful to the enemy? All of us are manipulative to some degree. Isn't positive manip-ulation common?"
- *Shallow emotions*—"Anger can lead to being labeled a psychopath."
- *Impulsive*—"Can be associated with creativity, living in the now, being spontaneous and free."
- *Poor behavioral controls*—"Violent and aggressive outbursts may be a defensive mechanism, a false front, a tool for survival in a jungle."
- *Need for excitement*—"Courage to reject the routine, monoto-nous, or uninteresting. Living on the edge, doing things that are risky, exciting, challenging, living life to its fullest, being alive rather than dull, boring, and almost dead."
- *Lack of responsibility*—"Shouldn't focus on human weak-nesses that are common."

• *Early behavior problems* and *adult antisocial behavior*—''Is a criminal record reflective of badness or nonconformity?''

Interestingly, he had nothing to say about *Lack of remorse or guilt.*

In a recent article for *The New York Times,* Daniel Goleman wrote, ''Data suggest that in general about 2 to 3 percent of people are estimated to be psychopaths—with the rate twice as high among those who live in the fragmented families of the inner cities.''[9] However, this statement, and others proclaiming an increase of psychopathy in our society, confuses criminality and social deviance with psychopathy.

While crime—and the socially deviant behavior that helps to but doesn't completely define psychopathy—is already high among the lower class, and is rising in society as a whole, we don't know if the relative number of psychopaths among us is also on the increase. Sociobiologists take the view that behavior development is influenced by genetic factors, and they might argue that the number of psychopaths *must* be increasing, simply because they are very promiscuous and produce large numbers of children, some of whom may inherit a predisposition for psychopathy.

I'll examine this argument and its chilling implications in later chapters on the roots of psychopathy. Before doing so, however, it is necessary to discuss the *known* aspects of the enigma. The next step into the heart of the matter brings us to the role of conscience in the regulation of behavior.

Chapter 5

Internal Controls: The Missing Piece

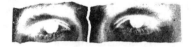

When a rogue kisses you, count your teeth.
—Hebrew proverb

Elyse met Jeffrey in the summer of 1984, and she was never to forget that day. She was at the beach with some friends when she spied him and was completely charmed by his huge, bright smile. He walked right up to her and asked for her phone number, and his effrontery somehow disarmed her—she just gave in to his smile and his utter lack of self-consciousness. He called her the next day and then somehow showed up at her job. So it began . . . with a smile.

She was working at a daycare center then. Jeffrey began meeting her at work for her coffee breaks, then for her lunch breaks, for her bus rides home; every time she walked out of the building, Jeffrey was there waiting. He told her very little about himself—said he was a cartoonist trying to get his own strip. Sometimes he carried large amounts of cash; at other times he was dead broke and used her money. He didn't live anywhere in particular, and all his clothes were "borrowed." He was funny—hilarious, Elyse thought. When it was all over, she realized that the humor had been both the draw and the distraction. The whole time he had been cannibalizing her life, she'd been laughing her head off at his jokes.

He talked nonstop, describing all his ideas, schemes, and plans, but none ever amounted to anything. Whenever she asked him about some plan he'd described, he seemed annoyed. "Oh, *that!* I'm onto something much bigger, *much* bigger now."

One day while they were at lunch, he was suddenly arrested. The next day Elyse went to visit him in jail. The police said he'd spent the night at a friend's house and the next day had sold the man's camera equipment. She didn't believe it, but the judge did. It turned out that Jeffrey was wanted by the police on a number of matters. Jeffrey went to prison.

Despite his incarceration he never lost his grip on Elyse. He wrote to her from prison at least once every day, sometimes as many as three times. He wrote of his talents, his dreams, his plans. He wrote of her and the life they would have together. He nearly drowned Elyse in words—"verbal vomit" was the phrase one writer used in describing a similar case. If only Jeffrey could find the right channel for his energies, he'd be on top of the world, he'd be able to do *anything,* he claimed. And he would give her the life she deserved—he loved her so much. She was so dazzled that the phrase "send money" at the end of one of his letters didn't even faze her.

In eight months Jeffrey was out. He went directly to Elyse's house and dazzled her anew, but her roommates were not impressed. Jeffrey propositioned one roommate and crawled into bed with the other while she slept. In the latter incident, he forced the young woman's shoulders down and held her fast, seeming to enjoy the fear on her face as he kept her from escaping. Needless to say, with Jeffrey in the house night and day, the communal living arrangement collapsed.

It was soon clear that he had no intention of leaving and no intention of finding a job. Still, Elyse kept trying to find work for him. The first interview he had was successful, but his first day on the job he stole all the money out of the cash register and disappeared for five days. Then a friend called to tell Elyse that Jeffrey was dealing drugs. When he showed up, light-hearted and talking a mile a minute, she confronted him. He denied all wrongdoing. And she believed him. She was on a yo-yo of believing, disbelieving, and believing again.

Elyse's parents stepped in and insisted that she consult a psychiatrist—they were fearful of her relationship with Jeffrey. They were immune to his charm and referred often to his "strange, flat eyes." But the psychiatrist was not so wary. He found Jeffrey "optimistic," "upbeat," "quite a character." Somehow, seeing the doctor taken in opened Elyse's eyes. She decided to break it off with Jeffrey then and there. Out on the street, she told him it was over. He grabbed her arm and stared her in the eye. "I'll never let you go, you know," he insisted, and she suddenly had a glimmer of what her parents meant about his eyes. "I'm always going to be with you, Elyse."

Within days she moved to another apartment—and Jeffrey began to stalk her.

Messages reached her—he'd kill himself if she didn't see him, he'd never let up until she did. But then the messages changed. Jeffrey wasn't going to kill himself; he was going to kill Elyse. Soon afterward he found her, broke down the door to her apartment, and grabbed her by her hair. Fortunately, her brother had decided to come over early from work and walked in just in time. At the sight of her brother, Jeffrey calmed down instantly. He smiled, said a casual hello, and left the apartment.

And that was that—the storm was over. He never came back. For years afterward Elyse got reports that Jeffrey had been arrested, mostly for robbery and fraud, once for assault. He went to jail; he got out and worked on a fishing boat for a while. The last she heard, he was back in prison for a long term. Often she wondered how she could have trusted him so completely from the beginning.

She never came up with an answer, and the knowledge of how close she had come to being swallowed up by Jeffrey's charm and then his anger kept her on guard with the men she met for a very long time.

Elyse, a former student of mine, now knows a lot about psychopaths, from both personal experience and formal training. But she still finds it difficult to understand how people like Jeffrey can so easily worm their way into someone's life and then simply move on. "For him," she said, "the rules of behavior were written in pencil, and he had a big eraser."

EVER SINCE THE release of the book and the movie, *The Silence of the Lambs,* reporters and television interviewers have been asking me if Hannibal "the Cannibal" Lecter, the terrifying central figure who is both a brilliant psychiatrist and a cannibalistic murderer, provides us with an accurate picture of the psychopath.

Clearly, as portrayed, Lecter has many of the characteristics of the psychopath. He is egocentric, grandiose, callous, manipulative, and remorseless. But he also seems more than a bit crazy. This is not surprising, given that both Lecter and the serial killer in the movie, Buffalo Bill, a transvestite who skins his female victims, bear some resemblance to a real-life psychotic serial killer, Edward Gein.

The head of the psychiatric hospital for the criminally insane in which Lecter is housed said, "Oh, he is a monster. A pure psychopath. So rare to capture one alive."

This is of course a grossly inaccurate statement, one that reflects the common assumption that all psychopaths are grisly serial killers who torture and maim for kicks. If Lecter *is* a psychopath, he is far from a typical one. If he did exist—he's a fictional character, after all—he would be a member of a rather select club. Serial killers are *extremely* rare; there are probably fewer than one hundred in North America. In contrast, there may be as many as 2 or 3 million psychopaths in North America. Even if almost all serial killers were psychopaths, this would mean that *for every psychopath who is a serial killer, there are 20,000 or 30,000 psychopaths who do not commit serial murder.*

In other words, portrayals of psychopaths that focus on grotesque and sadistic killers such as Lecter give the public a highly distorted view of the disorder. In most instances it is egocentricity, whim, and the promise of instant gratification for more commonplace needs, not the drooling satisfaction of bizarre power trips and sexual hungers, that motivate the psychopath to break the law.

Breaking the Rules

Society has many rules, some formalized in laws and others consisting of widely accepted beliefs about what is right and wrong. Each protects us as individuals and strengthens society's fabric. Fear of punishment certainly helps to keep us in line, but there are other reasons why we follow the rules:

- a rational appraisal of the odds of being caught

- a philosophical or theological idea of good and evil

- an appreciation of the need for social cooperation and harmony

- a capacity for thinking about, and being moved by, the feelings, rights, needs, and well-being of those around us

Learning to behave according to the rules and regulations of society, called socialization, is a complex process. On a practical level it teaches children "how things are done." In the process, socialization—through parenting, schooling, social experiences, religious training, and so forth—helps to create a system of beliefs, attitudes, and personal standards that determine how we interact with the world around us. Socialization also contributes to the formation of what most people call their conscience, the pesky inner voice that helps us to resist temptation and to feel guilty when we don't. Together, this inner voice and the internalized norms and rules of society act as an "inner policeman," regulating our behavior even in the absence of the many *external* controls, such as laws, our perceptions of what others expect of us, and real-life policemen. It's no overstatement to say that our internal controls make society work. Our collective amazement and fascination with the psychopath's utter disregard for rules suggests, by comparison, the power our "inner policemen" actually have over us.

However, for psychopaths like Jeffrey, the social experiences that normally build a conscience never take hold. Such people don't have an inner voice to guide them; they *know* the rules but follow only those they choose to follow, no matter what the repercussions for others. They have little resistance to temptation, and their transgressions elicit no guilt. Without the shackles of a nagging conscience, they feel free to satisfy their needs and wants and do whatever they think they can get away with. Any antisocial act, from petty theft to bloody murder, becomes possible.

We don't know why the conscience of the psychopath—if it exists at all—is so weak. However, we can make some reasonable guesses:

- Psychopaths have little aptitude for experiencing the emotional responses—fear and anxiety—that are the mainsprings of conscience.[1]

In most people, early childhood punishment produces lifelong links between social taboos and feelings of anxiety. The anxiety associated with potential punishment for an act helps to suppress the act. In fact, anxiety may help to suppress even the *idea* of the act: "I considered taking the money but I quickly put the thought out of my mind."

But in psychopaths, the links between prohibited acts and anxiety are weak, and the threat of punishment fails to deter them. Perhaps for this reason, Jeffrey's record of arrests and convictions looked like the criminal history of an amnesiac: No punishment ever had the slightest effect in dissuading him from gratifying his impulses.

PSYCHOPATHS ARE VERY good at giving their undivided attention to things that interest them most and at ignoring other things. Some clinicians have likened the process to a narrow-beam searchlight that focuses on only one thing at a time. Others suggest that it is similar to the concentration with which a predator stalks its prey.

This unusual ability to focus attention may or may not be a good thing, depending on the situation. For example, star athletes typically attribute much of their success to the power of concentration. A batter who takes his eye off the ball to watch a bird fly by, or who is momentarily distracted when someone shouts his name, is unlikely to improve his batting average.

On the other hand, many situations are complex and require that we pay attention to several things at the same time. If we concentrate on only what we find most interesting, we may miss something else of importance, perhaps a danger signal. This is what psychopaths often do: They pay so much attention to obtaining rewards and enjoying themselves that they ignore signals that could warn them of danger.

For example, some psychopaths earned reputations for being fearless fighter pilots during World War II, staying on their targets like terriers on an ankle. Yet, these pilots often failed to keep track of such unexciting details as fuel supply, altitude, location, and the position of other planes. Sometimes they became heroes, but more often they were killed or became known as opportunists, loners, or hotshots who couldn't be relied on—except to take care of themselves.

- The "inner speech" of psychopaths lacks emotional punch.

Conscience depends not only on the ability to imagine consequences but on the capacity to mentally "talk to oneself." Soviet psychologist A. R. Luria, for example, has shown that internalized speech—the inner voice—plays a crucial role in regulating behavior.[2]

But when psychopaths talk to themselves they are simply "reading lines." When Jeffrey attempted to rape Elyse's roommate, he may have thought to himself, "Shit. If I do this there'll be hell to pay. Maybe I'll get AIDS, she'll get pregnant, or Elyse will kill me." But if these thoughts *did* run through his mind they would have had about the same emotional impact on him if he'd thought, "Maybe I'll watch the ball game tonight." So, he never seriously considered the effect of his self-gratifying behavior on any of the people involved, including himself.

- Psychopaths have a weak capacity for mentally "picturing" the consequences of their behavior.[3]

Concrete rewards are pitted against vague future consequences—with the rewards clearly the stronger contender. The mental image of the consequences *for the victim* are particularly fuzzy. So, Jeffrey saw in Elyse not a companion but rather a "connection"—a supplier of shelter, clothing, food, money, recreation, and sexual gratification. The consequences *to her* of his actions didn't even enter his consciousness. When it became clear that he'd squeezed all he could out of his association with her, he simply moved on to another source of goodies.

They Pick and Choose

Of course, psychopaths are not *completely* unresponsive to the myriad rules and taboos that hold society together. After all, they are not automatons, blindly responding to momentary needs, urges, and opportunities. It is just that they are much freer than the rest of us to pick and choose the rules and restrictions they will adhere to.

For most of us even the *imagined* threat of criticism functions to control our behavior. We are haunted to some degree by questions about our self-worth. As a consequence, we continually attempt to prove to ourselves and others that we are okay people, credible, trustworthy, and competent.

In sharp contrast, the psychopath carries out his evaluation of a situation—what he will get out of it and at what cost—without the usual anxieties, doubts, and concerns about being humiliated, causing pain, sabotaging future plans, in short, the infinite possibilities that people of conscience consider when deliberating possible actions. For those of us who have been successfully socialized, imagining the world as the psychopath experiences it is close to impossible.

RUNNING PARALLEL TO the seawall in West Vancouver where I do my jogging is a railway track, used only a few times a day. About a year ago the signals controlling the car-crossing were activated and traffic began to back up. I had just finished my run and was cooling off nearby. It soon became clear to me that although the signals continued to flash, they had malfunctioned and no train was coming. However, the car at the front of the line did not move, even after most of the other cars began to pull around it. When I left about ten minutes later, the signal lights were still flashing and the first car still hadn't budged.

Think about the driver of that car and the psychopath as occupying opposite ends of a continuum of internal restraint. The former slavishly follows the rules, and the latter simply ignores them. One passively accepts the supreme authority of the inner voice that says "no"; the other tells it to "get lost."

This inner voice presents problems for those whose beliefs put them in conflict with society. As a piece of graffiti written during the French student revolts of 1968 put it, "There is a sleeping cop in all of us. He must be killed."

Psychocinema

The public's fascination with the smooth con artist and the cold-blooded killer, unbounded by the dictates of society and conscience, has never been stronger. *Goodfellas, Misery, Pacific Heights, Sleeping with the Enemy, In Broad Daylight, Love, Lies, and Murder, Small Sacrifices, Cape Fear, In a Child's Name*, and the particularly explicit chiller *The Silence of the Lambs*, are just a few of the most popular movies at this writing. True and reenacted crime shows, such as *Hard Copy, A Current Affair*, and *America's Most Wanted*, are now a television staple.

Bruce Weber, in a February 10, 1991, *New York Times* article called "Cozying Up to the Psychopath That Lurks Deep Within," reminded us that the story-teller's fascination with "the perversely twisted mind" is nothing new: "From Iago to Norman Bates, Dr. Jekyll to Harry Lime, Vladimir Nabakov's Humbert Humbert to David Lynch's Leland Palmer/Bob, the logic of villainy has been fictionally explored, on the page, the stage and the screen, over and over. Even when failed by their powers of sheer imagining, writers and actors have drawn inspiration from grim reality: Jack the Ripper, Lizzie Borden, Dick and Perry, Gary Gilmore, Charles Manson, not to mention Adolf Hitler, Joseph Stalin and Richard III. By now, Saddam Hussein is undoubtedly a twinkle in some wordsmith's eye."

The question is, Why? What accounts for the terrific power that the personality without conscience has over our collective imagination? "Clearly, evil is alluring," wrote Weber, "and not just to those who would dramatize it. From mild naughtiness to vicious criminality, the performance of bad deeds is something the rest of the population evidently wants to know about. This is one way to explain why the psychopath, that personification of remorseless evildoing, has such an established place in the public consciousness."

Weber pursued this line of thought with forensic psychiatrist Ronald Markman, who (along with Dominick Bosco) wrote *Alone with the Devil*, a book about Markman's professional work with murderers. The psychiatrist suggested that as an audience we identify with psychopaths, living out our fantasies of life with no internal controls. "There is something inside them that is also inside us and we are attracted to them so we can find out what that something is," Markman wrote. In Weber's interview he went even further: "We're all psychopaths under the skin."

Psychiatrist Joanne Intrator, at the Mount Sinai Medical Center in New York, offers a course titled The Psychopath in Fact and Film, in which she explains how film lends itself to this form of indentification, raising moviegoing from a level of casual curiosity to an act of emotionally charged voyeurism. She said that cinema "allows us to slip easily into the vicarious pleasure of the voyeur. A darkened room subdues our conscious moral world and allows us another focus of an inner state not dominated by the constraints of superego [conscience]. In the dark we are enjoying, with a subtle consciousness, aggressive and sexual pleasure at seemingly no cost."[4]

These cinematic experiences may have a beneficial effect on psychologically healthy people, reminding them of the danger and destructiveness that psychopathy carries with it. On the other hand, these experiences may also serve as powerful role models for those with poorly developed internal standards, serious psychological problems, or feelings of alienation from mainstream society.

Rebel Without a Cause

In 1944, psychoanalyst Robert Lindner wrote a classic study of criminal psychopathy, *Rebel Without a Cause*.[5] Lindner viewed psychopathy as a plague, a terrible force whose destructive potential is greatly underestimated. He described psychopaths in terms of their relationship to society:

> The psychopath is a rebel, a religious disobeyer of prevailing codes and standards . . . a rebel without a cause, an agitator without a slogan, a revolutionary without a program; in other words, his rebelliousness is aimed to achieve goals satisfactory to him alone; he is incapable of exertions for the sake of others. All his efforts, under no matter what guise, represent investments designed to satisfy his immediate wishes and desires. [p. 2]

The culture may change but the psychopathic "rebel" remains the same. In the mid-1940s, Lindner wrote that psychopaths were often to be found at the edges of society where they "sparkle with the glitter of personal freedom, the checks and reins of the community are absent and there are no limits either in a physical or in a psychological sense." [p. 13]

Today the psychopath appears to be everywhere among us, and we must ask ourselves some important questions. Why is our fascination with psychopathy growing—in our movies, on television, in our mass market books and magazines? Why are more and more crimes of violence being committed by young people? And what is it about our society that leads one expert to say:

> The young criminal you see today is more detached from his victim, more ready to hurt or kill. The lack of empathy for their victims among young criminals is just one symptom of a problem that afflicts the whole society. The general stance of the psychopath is more common these days; the

sense that I am responsible for the well-being of others is on the wane.[6]

Are we unknowingly allowing a society to evolve that is the perfect breeding ground, and perhaps even a "killing field," for psychopaths? As our morning newspaper tells us, this question grows more pressing every day.

Chapter 6

Crime: The Logical Choice

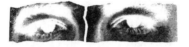

If crime is the job description, the psychopath is the perfect applicant.

In Fritz Lang's classic 1931 movie *M*, Peter Lorre played a
child molester/murderer who snatches his unlucky victims off
the streets as the impulse hits him. The police are unable to find
the killer, and the underworld of hoods and criminals takes on the
job itself. Once it tracks down its prey, the seedy, creepy outlaw
mob drags him to a deserted brewery and tries and convicts
him in its own underworld court. This movie was one of the
most effective dramatizations ever of the notion of "honor
among thieves."

Is there honor among thieves? Scratch the surface of the average prison inmate and you'll find some sort of moral code—not
necessarily the code of mainstream society, but a moral code
nevertheless, with its own rules and proscriptions. These criminals, although at odds with some of the rules and values of
society at large, may still follow the rules of their group—a
neighborhood, extended family, or gang. So, to be a criminal
does not mean to be without conscience—or even to be weakly
socialized. Criminals come to crime in a variety of ways, most
of them entailing outside forces:[1]

83

• Some criminals *learn* to do crime—they are raised in families or social environments in which criminal behavior, to one degree or another, is the accepted norm. One of our subjects, for example, had a father who was a "professional" thief and a mother who was a prostitute. From an early age he "went to work" with his father. More dramatic examples of these "subcultural criminals" include the mafia families and the bands of Gypsies common in some parts of Europe.

• Some criminals can be understood as largely the products of what is known as "the cycle of violence." Evidence is emerging to show that victims of early sexual, physical, or emotional abuse frequently become perpetrators of the same as adults. It is not uncommon, for example, to find that child molesters were themselves sexually abused, or for wife assaulters to have witnessed domestic violence at an early age.

• Still others run afoul of the law because of a powerful need—for example, drug addicts or people without skills or resources who buck their consciences and turn to robbery out of desperation. Many of the subjects in our research first began their criminal activities as refugees from broken, impoverished, or abusive homes; they turned to drugs for comfort or relief, and to crime to support their habit.

Others wound up as offenders by committing "crimes of passion." One of our subjects, a forty-year-old man without a criminal record or a history of violence, found some condoms in his wife's purse, got into a heated argument with her, "went crazy," and severely beat her. He received a sentence of two years but is certain to get an early parole.

For many of these individuals, negative social factors—poverty, family violence, child abuse, poor parenting, economic stress, alcohol and drug abuse, to name but a few—were contributors to, or even the cause of, their criminality. Indeed, had these factors *not* been present, many of these criminals would not have turned to crime.

But some individuals commit crime simply because it pays, it's easier than working, or it's exciting.[2] Not all are psychopaths, but for those who are, crime is less the result of adverse social conditions than of a character structure that operates with no reference to the rules and regulations of society. Typical of many of our psychopathic subjects, when asked why she committed crime a female in one of our studies replied, "You want the truth? Just for the fun of it."

Unlike most other criminals, psychopaths show no loyalty to groups, codes, or principles, other than to "look out for number one." Law enforcement agencies often make use of this when trying to solve a crime or to break up a gang or terrorist cell. To say, "Be smart, save your own skin; tell us who else was involved and you walk," is more likely to pay off with a psychopath than with an ordinary criminal.

TERRENCE MALICK'S MOVIE *Badlands*, loosely based on the killing career of Charles Starkweather and his girlfriend, Caril Ann Fugate, is a chilling film fantasy with a coldly realistic core. The fantasy resides in the character of Kit Carruthers, whose irresistible charm and slick patter is absolutely consistent with the psychopathic profile but whose attachment to his girlfriend Holly runs too deep and strong to ring true. One might be tempted to dismiss this movie as the typical Hollywood romance of the psychopath with a heart of gold, but look again. Behind Kit sits Holly, strictly along for the ride. It takes a second viewing for the real case history to pop into the foreground: If Kit is the moviemaker's conception of a psychopath, Holly is the real thing, a true "other" brilliantly portrayed by Sissy Spacek as a talking mask.

Two aspects of Holly's character exemplify and dramatize important aspects of the psychopathic personality. One is her emotional impoverishment and the clear sense she conveys of simply going through the motions of feeling deeply. One clue is the sometimes outrageous inappropriateness of her behavior. After Kit guns down her father before her eyes for objecting to his presence in Holly's life, the fifteen-year-old youngster slaps Kit's face. Later she flops into a chair and complains of a headache; later still she flees with Kit on a cross-country killing spree after he sets fire to her house to conceal her father's body.

In another example, with several more murders to his name

now, Kit lazily separates a terrified couple from their car at gunpoint and directs them out into an empty field. Casually, Holly falls into step with the frightened woman. "Hi," she says in her flat, childish voice. "What will happen?" asks the woman, desperate for some understanding of what's going on. "Oh," answers Holly, "Kit says he feels like he just might explode. I feel like that myself sometimes. Don't you?" The scene ends with Kit locking the two in a root cellar in the middle of the field. Just about to walk away, he suddenly shoots into the cellar door. "Think I got 'em?" he asks, as if swatting at flies in the dark.

Perhaps the film's most subtle evidence of psychopathy comes through in Holly's narration of the film, delivered in a monotone and embellished with phrases drawn straight from the glossies telling young girls what they should feel. Holly speaks of the love she and Kit share, but the actress manages somehow to convey the notion that Holly has no experiential knowledge of the feelings she reports. If there was ever an example of "knowing the words but not the music," Spacek's character is it, giving viewers a firsthand experience of the odd sensation, the unnamable distrust and skin-crawling feeling, that many—lay people and professionals alike—report after their interactions with psychopaths.

The Formula for Crime

In many respects it is difficult to see how *any* psychopaths—with their lack of internal controls, their unconventional attitudes about ethics and morality, their callous, remorseless, and egocentric view of the world, and so forth—could manage to avoid coming into conflict with society at some point in their lives. A great many do, of course, and their criminal activities cover the spectrum of possibilities, from petty theft and embezzlement to assault, extortion, and armed robbery, from vandalism and disturbing the peace to kidnapping, murder, and crimes against the state such as treason, espionage, and terrorism.

Although not all criminals are psychopaths, and not all psychopaths are criminals, psychopaths are well represented in our prison populations and are responsible for crime far out of proportion to their numbers:[3]

- On average, about 20 percent of male and female prison inmates are psychopaths.
- Psychopaths are responsible for more than 50 percent of the serious crimes committed.

The truth is, the personality structure of the psychopath spells trouble for the rest of us. Just as the great white shark is a natural killing machine, psychopaths naturally slip into the role of criminal. Their readiness to take advantage of any situation that arises, combined with their lack of the internal controls we know as conscience, creates a potent formula for crime.

So, for example, when a dazzling smile throws a young woman on the beach off guard, a young psychopath like Jeffrey wastes no time in attaching himself firmly and finding ways of drawing off all the warmth, sexual gratification, shelter, food, and money he can—all in the name of "love."

When a young man of the age and type that appeals to John Wayne Gacy happens to apply for a job at his business, Gacy wastes no time in intimidating the boy into sex play. And he doesn't stop until he murders the boy and disposes of his body underneath his house.[4]

When Utah killer Gary Gilmore has an argument with his girlfriend, he drives around (with another woman) until the urge to vent his rage becomes too great to contain. He pulls into a gas station, leaves his young companion alone to listen to the radio for a few minutes, and shoots to death the first person he comes across. The next night he repeats the pattern. He describes the two men he shoots as simply being in the wrong place at the wrong time, in the way of his need to strike out.[5]

A recent study by the FBI found that 44% of the offenders who killed a law enforcement officer on duty were psychopaths. [*Killed in the Line of Duty*, The Uniform Crime Reports Section, Federal Bureau of Investigation, United States Department of Justice, September, 1992]

Living for the Moment

Although a student of New Age philosophies might shudder at the desecration of sacred principles, much of the psychopath's behavior and motivation makes sense if we think of him or her as a person rooted completely in the present and unable to resist a good opportunity. As an inmate who scored high on the *Psychopathy Checklist* said, "What's a guy gonna do? She had a nice ass. I helped myself." He was convicted of rape. Another was picked up by police after he appeared on a television game show in the very city where his victims lived. Five minutes of stardom and two years in prison!

In the *Playboy* interview shortly before his execution, Gary Gilmore conveyed a sense of what it was like to be anchored so firmly in the present. When asked why, although he had a very high IQ, he had been caught at crime so often, Gilmore responded:

> I got away with a couple of things. I ain't a great thief. I'm impulsive. Don't plan, don't think. You don't have to be super intelligent to get away with that shit, you just have to think. But I don't. I'm impatient. Not greedy enough. I could have gotten away with lots of things that I got caught for. I don't, ah, really understand it. Maybe I quit caring a long time ago.[6]

Psychopathic Violence —Cold-blooded and "Casual"

Even more troubling than their heavy involvement in crime is the evidence that both male and female psychopaths are much more likely to be *violent* and *aggressive* than are other individuals.[7] Of course, violence is not uncommon in most offender populations, but psychopaths still manage to stand out. They commit more than twice as many violent and aggressive acts, both in and out of prison, as do other criminals.

Troubling, yes, but not surprising. While most of us have

strong inhibitions about physically injuring others, psychopaths typically do not. For them, violence and threats are handy tools to be used when they are angered, defied, or frustrated, and they give little thought to the pain and humiliation experienced by the victims. Their violence is callous and instrumental—used to satisfy a simple need, such as sex, or to obtain something he or she wants—and the psychopath's reactions to the event are much more likely to be indifference, a sense of power, pleasure, or smug satisfaction than regret at the damage done. Certainly nothing to lose any sleep over.

Compare the psychopath's reactions with those of law enforcement officers compelled to use deadly force in the line of duty. Unlike the fictional characters in movies who can kill ten bad guys before dinner and still have seconds—"Dirty Harry" Callahan, played by Clint ("Make my day") Eastwood, comes to mind—most police officers are severely disturbed by shootings, and many experience "emotional flashbacks" or suffer from what has come to be known as *posttraumatic stress syndrome.* The aftereffects can be so debilitating that many jurisdictions routinely stipulate that any officer involved in a shooting, fatal or not, must receive psychological counseling.

Such counseling would be wasted on psychopaths. Even experienced and case-hardened professionals find it unnerving when they see a psychopath's reaction to a gut-wrenching event or listen to him or her casually describe a brutal offense as if an apple had been peeled or a fish gutted.

• Gary Gilmore, in explaining to his interviewers how he came to have the nickname "Hammersmith" in prison, offers a good example of the psychopath's uninhibited approach to violence.[8] A friend of Gilmore's, LeRoy, was robbed and beaten up in prison. He sent word to Gilmore that he needed help in getting even with the perpetrator, Bill. "That night I caught Bill sitting down watching a football game," recounts Gilmore, "and I just planted the hammer in his head, turned around and walked off . . . How bad did I hurt him! [laughs] . . . they just kept me in the hole for four months and took Bill to Portland for brain surgery. But Bill was pretty fucked up anyhow. So, to answer your question, this guy nicknamed me Hammersmith over that. He gave me a little toy hammer to wear on a chain . . ." Apparently, Gilmore later claimed to have killed Bill with the hammer and to have committed another violent murder as well. The interviewers asked him, "Why did you go around telling everybody that you'd killed them? Were you bragging or confessing?"

Gilmore: "[laughing] More bragging, probably, to tell you the truth."

• An ex-con, previously diagnosed by a prison psychiatrist as a psychopath, calmly told the police that he had stabbed another man in a bar because the man refused his request to vacate a table. His explanation: He was cultivating a don't-mess-with-me image at the time and the victim had defied him in front of the other bar patrons.

ON NEW YEAR'S Day 1990, twenty-six-year-old Roxanne Murray killed her forty-two-year-old husband of five years with a 12-gauge shotgun. She told police she loved her husband but had to kill him. The court agreed, and the charge of second-degree murder was dropped.

The husband, Doug (Juicer) Murray, was a "pseudo-biker" with a "need for powerful motorcycles and weak, compliant women, and dogs—all possessions to be controlled." Over the years he had been charged with a string of rapes and assaults, none of which went to trial, for lack of witnesses. He had been married several times before and typically terrorized and battered the women he was involved with. In a macabre twist, "he once ran a home for sexually abused teens. He exploited them mentally and physically as he exploited most women, frequently taking compromising photographs for later use."

When Roxanne complained about the food bills for their fourteen dogs, Doug dragged her into the trailer, smashed her in the head with a loaded pistol, and shot her favorite dog in front of her. "That could happen to you," he told her. He "seemed incapable of sex without violence or absolute control. Fellatio was something to be demanded anywhere at any time or a beating followed. He forced his women into brutal fantasy rape scenarios. He forced several to play Russian roulette with a live round in each chamber." Roxanne's best friend said that "it

> was like Doug had several sides to him. Some of them were good, or he wanted to portray them as good, and some of them were just the worst that you could imagine."
>
> It seems that in pursuing his own brutal course Doug inadvertently helped the community to draw a line in the sand marking out the limits beyond which abused and terrorized victims are justified in taking drastic action to protect themselves. [from an article by Ken McQueen, *The Vancouver Sun*, March 1, 1991]

• An offender who scored high on the *Psychopathy Checklist* killed an elderly man during the course of a burglary, and casually gave this account of the affair: "I was rummaging around when this old geezer comes down stairs and . . . uh . . . he starts yelling and having a fucking fit . . . so I pop him one in the, uh, head and he still doesn't shut up. I give him a chop to the throat and he . . . like . . . staggers back and falls on the floor. He's gurgling and making sounds like a stuck pig [laughs] and he's really getting on my fucking nerves so I . . . uh . . . boot him a few times in the head. That shut him up . . . I'm pretty tired by now, so I grab a few beers from the fridge and turn on the TV and fall asleep. The cops woke me up [laughs]."

Such simple, dispassionate displays of violence are quite distinct from an act of violence exploding from a heated argument, a staggering emotional blow, uncontrollable anger, rage, or fear. Examples abound in the news media. And most people know what it is like to "lose it," sometimes with violent results, and to be appalled at their own actions. As I was writing this chapter, a sixty-five-year-old man with no criminal record was tried for attempted murder; he stabbed his ex-wife and her lawyer with a pocketknife during an extremely emotional child-custody hearing. A local psychiatrist testified that the man was so overwrought that he lost control, "went on automatic," and didn't even remember what he had done. The man, horrified at his actions, was acquitted.

Even had he been convicted he would have been a good bet for early parole. As criminologists have pointed out, homicides that occur when emotions run high during domestic disputes or arguments among friends or acquaintances are usually "onetime things," committed by otherwise upstanding, remorseful individuals and unlikely to be repeated.

The violence of psychopaths, however, lacks normal emotional "coloring" and is likely to be precipitated by everyday events. In a recent study we examined police reports describing the circumstances surrounding the most recent violent offenses committed by a sample of male criminals, about half of whom were psychopaths.[9] The violent crimes committed by the psychopaths and the other criminals differed in several important ways:

- The violence of the other criminals usually occurred during a domestic dispute or a period of intense emotional upheaval, but:

- The violence of the psychopaths frequently occurred during commission of a crime or during a drinking bout, or was motivated by revenge or retribution.

- Two-thirds of the victims of the other criminals were female family members, friends, or acquaintances, but:

- Two-thirds of the victims of the psychopaths were male strangers.

In general, psychopathic violence tends to be callous and cold-blooded, and more likely to be straightforward, uncomplicated, and businesslike than an expression of deep-seated distress or understandable precipitating factors. It lacks the "juice" or powerful emotion that accompanies the violence of most other individuals.

Perhaps the scariest aspect of psychopathic violence is the influence it has on the nature of violence in our urban centers. Muggings, drug deals gone bad, "wildings," aggressive panhandling, gang activities, "swarming," and attacks on designated target groups such as gays usually involve the dispassionate or unprovoked use of violence against strangers or victims of convenience. One of the models of this new wave of violence is the psychopathic thug portrayed in movies and television: "Nothing personal," he says as he goes about his business of violent self-indulgence. As a fifteen-year-old girl put it, "I see something I want so bad I just take it. The worst time, I pulled a knife on this girl, but I never hurt anybody. I just want things."[10]

A "NIGHTMARE" DRIVER plowed into a car and killed a mother and her small daughter. Witnesses reported that the driver "was rude and obnoxious after the accident. He was only concerned about it causing him to miss a date." In the ambulance with one of his victims, a badly injured two-month-old baby, the driver—who showed no evidence of alcohol or drug use—reportedly responded to the baby's cries with, "Can you shut the goddamn kid up?" [reported in *The Province*, Vancouver, April 25, 1990]

Sexual Violence

Rape provides a good example of the callous, selfish, and instrumental use of violence by psychopaths. Not all rapists are psychopaths, of course. Some rapists clearly are very disturbed individuals suffering from a variety of psychiatric and psychological problems. Others are the products of cultural and social attitudes that reduce women to subservient roles. The offenses of these men, although repugnant to society and horribly traumatic for the victims, may be more understandable than are those committed by psychopaths.

Perhaps half of the repeat or serial rapists are psychopaths.[11] Their acts are the result of a potent mixture: uninhibited expression of sexual drives and fantasies, desire for power and control, and perception of the victims as objects of pleasure or satisfaction. This mixture is well illustrated by John Oughton, called the "paper bag rapist" by the Vancouver press (he wore a paper bag over his head when he raped children and women). Oughton was diagnosed by a court psychiatrist as both a psychopath—"lacks a conscience, is manipulative, egocentric, untruthful, and lacks a capacity for love"—and a sexual sadist who "gets sexual excitement by inflicting psychological pressure on his victims."[12]

The Psychopath
as Wife Batterer

In recent years public awareness and intolerance of domestic violence have increased dramatically, resulting in aggressive prosecution and court-mandated treatment of offenders. Although the causes and dynamics of wife battering are complex and involve myriad economic, social, and psychological factors, there is some evidence that psychopaths constitute a significant proportion of persistent batterers.

In a recent study, we administered the *Psychopathy Checklist* to a sample of men taking part, either voluntarily or as part of a sentence, in a treatment program for wife assaulters.[13] We found that 25 percent of the men in the sample were psychopaths, a percentage similar to that found in prison populations. We don't know the percentage of psychopathic wife assaulters who do *not* enter treatment programs, but I suspect it is at least as high.

The suggestion that many of the men who continually assault their wives are psychopaths has serious ramifications for treatment programs. This is because the behavior of psychopaths is notoriously resistant to change (a topic I will discuss in a later chapter). The resources available to run programs for assaultive husbands usually are limited, and many treatment groups have long waiting lists. Psychopaths, more than other men, are likely to attend these programs simply to appease the courts rather than to change their behavior, and they may do little more than occupy a seat that could be better used by someone else.

Furthermore, psychopaths undoubtedly have disrupting effects on such programs. But perhaps the most disturbing consequence of sending a psychopath into such a therapy situation is the false sense of security it can engender in the assaulter's wife. "He's been treated. He should better now," she might conclude, thus missing the chance to end the abusive relationship.

MR. LEBLANC WAS convicted of assaulting his common-law wife and ordered by the court to attend a treatment group for assaultive husbands. Charming and amiable, he described the assault as a very minor—and yes, even unfortunate—altercation in which he struck out in anger during an argument with his wife. The police report, however, indicated that he had blackened her eyes and broken her nose, and that this assault was only the latest in a string of similar episodes involving many other women. In an interview prior to the start of his first treatment session he stated that he understood the problem and that all he needed was to learn some anger-management skills. He then proceeded to describe, in a pontificating way, the psychological dynamics and theories associated with family violence, and concluded that it was unlikely that the group could offer him much; however, he was willing to attend the sessions because he could help the other men gain some insight into their problems.

During the first session he casually commented that he had been a paratrooper in Vietnam, had received an MBA from Columbia University, and had started several successful business enterprises; details were sketchy. He said that his current offense was his first, and when the group leader pointed out that he had also received convictions for theft, fraud, and embezzlement, he smiled and said that they were all the result of petty misunderstandings.

He dominated the group discussions and spent most of his efforts in rather superficial, "pop psych" analyses of the other men. The group leader found him interesting, but most of the others were usually frustrated by his intellectual arrogance and aggressive manner. After a few sessions he dropped out of the group, and reportedly left the city, in clear violation of the court order against him. His claims to be a graduate of Columbia University and to have served in Vietnam turned out be false.

The Real Test: Can We Predict Their Behavior?

In capital murder cases in Texas, forensic psychiatrist James Grigson, "Dr. Death," routinely testifies that psychopathic murderers are *certain* to kill again.[14] As a result, there is no shortage of occupants for the cells on death row.

Grigson's certainty is offset by the belief, held by many clinicians and policy makers, that criminal behavior and violence *cannot* be predicted accurately.

As usual, the truth lies somewhere between these extremes. It doesn't take a genius to realize that people who have a history of criminality or violence are more dangerous than others. A good predictor of what someone will do in the future is what he or she has done in the past, a maxim that provides the basis for many of the decisions made by the criminal justice system.

Evidence from at least half a dozen recent studies clearly demonstrates that predictions about criminal and violent behavior can be improved considerably if we also know whether the individual is a psychopath, as defined by the *Psychopathy Checklist*.[15] These studies looked at the recidivism rates (commission of new offenses) of federal offenders following their release from prison. These studies show that, on average:

- The recidivism rate of psychopaths is about *double* that of other offenders.

- The *violent* recidivism rate of psychopaths is about *triple* that of other offenders.

An area of great concern to the public is the release on parole of sexual offenders. As I indicated earlier, it is important to distinguish between sexual offenders who are psychopaths and those who are not. The importance of this distinction for parole boards is highlighted by a recent study of rapists released from prison following an intensive treatment program.[16] Almost one-third of the released men raped again. For the most part, the repeat rapists had a high score on the *Psychopathy Checklist* and had shown, prior to release, evidence of deviant sexual arousal to depictions of violence, as measured by an electronic device placed around the penis. When used to predict which released offenders would rape again, these two variables—psychopathy and deviant arousal—were correct three times out of four.

Because of results like this, the criminal justice system is showing renewed interest in the association between psychopathy, recidivism, and violence. This interest is not confined to criminals about to be released from prison. For example, several forensic psychiatric hospitals now use the *Psychopathy Checklist* to help make decisions about the security level to which a patient should be assigned.[17]

Do They Grow Out of It?

Think about some relatives or friends you have known since childhood: the shy, inhibited girlfriend; the outgoing, gregarious brother; the fast-talking, sleazy cousin; the wild, hostile, aggressive neighbor. What were they like when they were ten years old?

Although people change, in some cases a great deal, many personality traits and behavioral patterns remain stable throughout life. For example, the boy who is afraid of his own shadow is more likely to become a timid, anxious adult than a tough and fearless fighter. This is not to say that our personalities and behaviors become tightly fixed early in life, or that growth, maturation, and experience are not powerful forces in determining what sort of adults we will become. But there is a certain degree of continuity in how we interact with our environment. With respect to criminality, for example, several researchers have shown that the childhood traits of timidity, restlessness, and aggressiveness are remarkably persistent, at least into early adulthood.[18]

It is not surprising, then, that the antisocial and criminal activities of adult psychopaths are continuations of behavior patterns that first showed themselves in childhood. But something interesting happens at the other end of the spectrum:[19]

- On average, the criminal activities of psychopaths remain at a high level until around age forty, after which they decrease sharply.

- This decrease is more dramatic for nonviolent offenses than for violent ones.

What accounts for the decrease in antisocial behavior that many psychopaths show in middle age? Several plausible explanations have been advanced: They "burn out," mature, get tired of being in prison or in conflict with the law, develop new strategies for beating the system, find someone who understands them, restructure their view of themselves and the world, and so on.

But before concluding that aging psychopaths pose little threat to society, consider the following:

- Not all psychopaths give up crime in middle age; many continue to commit offenses well into their senior years.

- A decrease in criminality does not necessarily mean that there has been a fundamental change in personality.

These are important points. Some psychopaths continue to commit offenses, especially violent ones, until the day they die. And research suggests that many of those whose criminal activities do decrease with age still have much the same core personality traits as those described in chapter 3—that is, they remain egocentric, shallow, manipulative, and callous. The difference is that they have learned to satisfy their needs in ways that are not as grossly antisocial as before. However, this does not mean that their behavior is now moral and ethical.

Thus, a woman whose "reformed" husband now manages to stay out of trouble with the law, cheats on her less regularly than before, and expresses love for her, may well wonder if her man has "really changed at all," particularly if she seldom knows where he is or what he is up to. If that man were a psychopath, I would very much doubt that he has changed.

AT AGE THIRTY-FIVE, a diagnosed psychopath with a lengthy record of criminal behavior and violence decided to turn her life around. She took a great many courses in prison and, following her release at age forty-two, obtained a university degree in counseling psychology. She began working with street kids and has not been charged with any offense during the past five years. Some people in the community consider her a success story. However, she has been dismissed from several jobs over the misuse of funds and making threats against her co-workers and supervisors. Because many people take the threats seriously and because they fear that publicity about her activities would embarrass them and their organizations, they have not taken formal action against her. Some of those who know her think she is an interesting woman whose criminal past was the result of unfavorable social conditions and bad luck; others think she is much the same person she always was—callous, arrogant, manipulative, egocentric—with the only discernible difference being that she now manages to remain out of contact with the law.

A Perfect Score

I will end this chapter with a brief account of an offender whom two independent assessors agreed should receive the maximum possible score on the *Psychopathy Checklist*, a score given to fewer than one in two hundred serious offenders.

Earl was a forty-year-old serving a three-year sentence for assault. Both assessors found the interview with him interesting, even exciting, for he exuded a captivating energy that kept them on the edge of their seats. At the same time, they were shocked and repelled by what he had to say and by the casual, matter-of-fact way in which he said it. As one of the assessors put it, "I was really fascinated by this guy, but he was from another planet. He scared the shit out of me!"

Earl came from a stable working-class family, the third of four children. His problems with society began early: In kindergarten he stabbed a teacher with a fork after she had forced him to sit in his seat; at age ten he was procuring young girls (including his twelve-year-old sister) for sexual favors for his older friends; and at age thirteen he was convicted for stealing from his parents and forging their names on checks. "Yeah, I spent a few months in juvey [a juvenile detention center], but I got away with a fucking lot more than they caught me for."

Since then, there is very little Earl hasn't done, most of it to other people. His record is littered with charges for robbery,

99

traffic violations, assault, rape, theft, fraud, unlawful confinement, pimping, and attempted murder. Yet, he has spent surprisingly little time in prison. In many cases the charges were dropped because the victim refused to testify, and in other cases because of lack of evidence or because Earl was able to come up with a convincing explanation for his behavior. Even when convicted, he typically managed to obtain early parole, seemingly inexplicable in view of his behavior in prison.

An entry in a psychological report tells the story: "The most salient thing about Earl is his obsession with absolute power. . . . He values people only insofar as they bend to his will or can be coerced or manipulated into doing what he wants. He constantly sizes up his prospects for exploiting people and situations." Other prison files describe how, in his quest for power and control, he walks a fine line between inmates and staff and is both feared and admired by both sides. He is very skilled in the use of threats, intimidation, muscle, bribery, and drugs, and he "regularly informs on other inmates in an effort to save his ass and to obtain privileges. The con code means nothing to him unless he personally gets something out of it."

His relations with women are as shallow and predatory as the rest of his behavior. He attests to having had several hundred live-in relationships, ranging from days to weeks, and an inestimable number of sexual contacts over the years. When asked how many children he has, Earl replied, "I don't really know. A few, I guess. I've been accused of being the father, but I'd say, 'Fuck you! How do I know it's mine?' " He routinely terrorized and assaulted the women in his life, sexually abused his daughter, and raped her girlfriend. His propensities for sadistic sexual behavior carry over into prison, where he is well known for his "aggressive homosexuality."

One of the most striking features of Earl's personality is his grandiosity; entries scattered through his files make reference to his dramatic, inflated, and pompous way of communicating. As one of my assessors wrote, "If I hadn't been so afraid of him I would have laughed in his face at his blatant self-worship." As Earl put it, "I'm always being told by others how great I am and how there's nothing I can't do—sometimes I think they're just shitting me, but a man's got to believe in himself, right? When I check myself out, I like what I see."

At the time of the interview, several years ago, Earl was being considered for parole. In his application to the parole board he had this to say: "I've matured a lot and don't see any future in prison life. I've got a lot to offer society, and I've worked hard analyzing my weaknesses and strengths. My goal is to be a good citizen, live modestly, and have a loving relationship with a good woman. I believe I've become more honest and trustworthy. My reputation is sacred to me." The interviewer commented, "The irony of the fact that Earl was widely known as a notorious bullshitter with dozens of aliases was not lost on me."

Surprisingly, the prison psychologist and psychiatrist thought that Earl *had* shown improvement during his current stay in prison, and on the basis of their dealings with him they considered him a good parole risk. But, as one of my interviewers said, "If even half of what he told me is true, he should never be let out." Earl was aware that our assessments were strictly confidential, conducted as part of a research project in which we were legally and ethically prevented from communicating our findings to the institutional authorities unless he actually threatened to harm himself or others. His persona with us therefore was more open than was the one he displayed in preparation for his parole application. As it turned out, Earl's parole was denied, and he began to accuse my interviewer of divulging what he had confided to him. The interviewer, fearing reprisal from Earl's friends on the outside, left on a prolonged trip to Europe and is now working in England. Earl was recently released from prison, and my interviewer has no plans to return to Canada in the near future.

Chapter **7**

White-Collar
Psychopaths

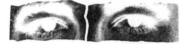

The faults of the burglar are the qualities of the financier.
—George Bernard Shaw, preface,
Major Barbara

In July 1987, in response to an article that appeared in *The New York Times* summarizing my work on psychopathy,[1] I received a letter from Assistant District Attorney (ADA) Brian Rosner of New York. He wrote that he had recently spoke at a sentencing hearing of a man who had been convicted of a multimillion-dollar international bank fraud. "Your words, as reported in the article, described this defendant to a 't.' . . . In the Frauds Bureau, our stock-in-trade is, to paraphrase your words, the shyster attorney, doctor and businessman. Your work, I think, will assist us in convincing courts to understand why educated men in three-piece suits commit crime and what must be done with them at sentencing. For your interest, I've enclosed some material from this case. If ever you needed facts to confirm a theory, here they are."[2]

This letter was accompanied by a package of materials describing the exploits of a thirty-six-year-old John Grambling, Jr., who, with the help of a cohort, defrauded not one or two but many banks into freely and confidently handing over millions of dollars, although the two had no collateral whatsoever. An article in the *Wall Street Journal* describing Grambling's career of fraud was headlined this way: BORROWING MILLIONS WITHOUT COLLATERAL TAKES INGENUITY, BUT JOHN GRAMBLING KNOWS HOW TO APPEAL TO BANKS AND HOW TO FAKE ASSETS.[3] The article opened with this:

> A couple of years back, two businessmen on the make tried to steal $36.5 million from four banks and a savings and loan association. And without pointing a gun at anybody, they actually made off with $23.5 million. Their batting average wasn't bad, but they got caught.

The scams rested almost completely on appearances. Between them, Grambling and his associate were able to convince a long line of officials in many lending institutions that they were men to be trusted. In fact, the two finessed an impressive credit rating, repaying one loan by floating another, and so on down the line.

In searching for an explanation of how such swindles occur, the *Journal* writer elicited these reactions from bankers:

- "Banks are highly competitive in trying to place good loans."

- Grambling's "very nice social graces" gave him credibility.

- A person intent upon fraud "is going to get it done."

- Grambling "should be compelled to wear a bell around his neck."

As the court transcripts and other legal papers in the package sent to me attest,[4] Grambling makes his living by using charm, deceit, and manipulation to gain the confidence of his victims. Although he may be able to offer plausible explanations for what he has done, it is clear from the documents and a recent book on the case written by Brian Rosner,[5] that John Grambling's reported behavior is compatible with the concept of psychopathy described in this book. At the very least, the story is a graphic morality tale about a breed of predators whose charming demeanor and anemic conscience grease the way for fleecing institutions and people—for what is euphemistically called white-collar crime. They have charming smiles on their faces and a trustworthy tone to their voices, but never—and this is a guarantee—do they wear warning bells around their necks.

For psychopaths who have an entrepreneurial bent, the Grambling case—and others like it—is a model for using education and social connections to separate people and institutions from their money without using violence. Unlike "ordinary" white-collar criminals, the deceit and manipulation of these individuals are not confined to simply making money; these qualities pervade their dealings with everyone and everything, including family, friends, and the justice system. They often manage to avoid prison, and even if caught and convicted they usually receive a light sentence and an early parole, only to continue where they left off.

Yet, their crimes have a devastating impact on society. Consider the following comments about Grambling, made by ADA Brian Rosner during the sentencing hearing:[6]

- The crimes of Grambling are calculated crimes of greed, driven by a lust to exercise power over the lives and fortunes of others. It is a lust often seen in the most vicious criminal. . . . The work of a man of incalculable evil. [p. 87]

- He has littered this nation with broken careers and aspirations. The monetary destruction he has caused can be calculated. The human suffering and psychological damage cannot. [p. 86]

- Though his tools are genteel, his instincts are as savage as the street brute. [p. 83]

In addition to bilking financial institutions, Grambling used the stationery of a prestigious accounting firm to forge financial statements that enabled him to get loans. At the same time, he conned the senior member of the firm—a philanthropy consultant—and his colleague into helping him establish a fraudulent charity for the elderly. To these two men, said Rosner, "Grambling is simply the smoothest con man they have ever met."[7]

> CHARMING PEOPLE LIVE up to the very edge of their charm, and behave just as outrageously as the world allows.
> —Logan Pearsall Smith, *Afterthoughts*, p. 3.

His crimes were not limited to faceless financial institutions. For example, he forged his sister-in-law's income tax form and tricked her into signing a mortgage note for $4.5 million. He kept the money and left her liable for the debt. On his arrest, she said that one can't imagine "the relief I felt when I knew he was behind bars. . . . The little people he's hurt. . . . God, he's not going to be able to hurt anybody now."[8]

His father-in-law wrote that Grambling expressed regret for his past errors, talked of his therapy, his "100% rehabilitation," and plans for making up for his sins, "all while *he was on his way to rip off another bank*."[9] While free on his own recognizance Grambling committed additional frauds, engaging in a "coast-to-coast crime wave."[10] His expressions of remorse were belied by his conduct.

And what did Grambling have to say about all this? Quite a bit, as it turns out. Some of his comments are revealing and worth presenting here as an example of a characteristic typically found in psychopaths: facile distortions of reality even when they *know* that others are aware of the facts. The comments are taken from a letter sent to the court in an attempt to obtain a light prison sentence, and from the proceedings of the sentencing hearing.

- I have developed through my training in finance into a financial architect. I am a builder. I am not a professional "con-man" or "scam-artist."[11]

- I never had a legal problem in any job I held prior to 1983, be it related to finance or any other field.[12]

- I am a very feeling person.[13]

As Grambling was well aware, his statements did not square with the facts available to the court. He *was* a "scam artist," he *did* have legal problems before 1983, and, by all reports, he was *not* a "feeling person" in the normal sense of the term. His scams and previous legal difficulties are well documented. As a university student in the early 1970s he embezzled several thousand dollars from his fraternity. Wishing to avoid a scandal, the fraternity accepted a check from Grambling's father and did not press charges.

In Grambling's first job, in a major investment banking house, his employer considered him a "professional incompetent," and he was "encouraged" to leave.[14] In a subsequent financial job he misrepresented the position he held and cheated the firm. Grambling was permitted to resign and went into business for himself as a forger and a thief.[15]

As for feelings, Rosner said of Grambling's wife, "She had a fear for her boys. Grambling had always been a poor father, emotionless and never available. He had lied to his sons about his crimes, just as he lied to anyone who asked. And he had lied to her, about too many things to be counted."[16] [p. 362] Further, "She never knew her husband: 'It's as if I went to bed with a boy scout, and woke up with Jack the Ripper.' She was as deceived as anyone. She has said that she wishes she had just been raped. Then it would be over with. . . . One friend, thinking he was being sympathetic, told her he could not understand why Grambling's sentence was so high for 'just a white-collar crime.' She could have ripped out the friend's throat. The 'just a white-collar crime' is something she lives with every day." [p. 390] And Rosner and his colleagues concluded, on the basis of an extensive report on Grambling's family relations, that they had never "seen a more comprehensive analysis of the white-collar criminal mind: the relentless drive to accumulate wealth; the use of people to obtain that end; the abandonment of all emotion and human attachment other than self-love." [p. 361]

Grambling's ability to rationalize his behavior is typical of the attitude that psychopaths have toward their victims. In addition to his wish to be "liked by everyone," his euphemistic view of himself as a "financial architect," and his "fear of losing face," he considered his crimes logical responses to frustration and pressure, or more the victim's fault than his own. "In Grambling's mind, anyone who is stupid enough to trust or believe him deserves the consequences," said Rosner.[17]

Trust-Mongers

Grambling was able to use his charm, social skills, and family connections to gain the trust of others. He was aided by the common expectation that certain classes of people presumably are trustworthy because of their social or professional credentials. For example, lawyers, physicians, teachers, politicians, counselors, and so forth, generally do not have to work to earn our trust; they have it by virtue of their positions. Our guard may go up when we deal with a used-car salesman or a telephone solicitor, but we often blindly entrust our assets and well-being to a lawyer, doctor, or investment counselor.

In most cases our trust is not misplaced, but the very fact that we are so willing to give it makes us easy prey for every opportunistic shark we encounter. Most dangerous of all—the "Jaws" of the trust-mongers—are psychopaths. Having obtained our trust, they betray it with stunning callousness.

One of our subjects—I'll call him Brad—a forty-year-old lawyer who scored high on the *Psychopathy Checklist*, provides a good example of a psychopath's use of his professional position to selfishly satisfy personal needs. Brad comes from a respected professional family, has a younger sister who is a lawyer, and is serving four years for fraud and breach of trust involving several million dollars. He took the money from the trust accounts of several clients and forged checks drawn on the bank accounts of his sister and parents. He said that he had only borrowed the money to cover a disastrous run of bad luck on the stock market and that it was his intention to "pay back every cent, with interest." In fact, Brad's reputation for fast living was well known: He had been married three times, drove a Porsche, had an expensive condo, used cocaine, and piled up huge gambling debts with local bookies. He was very adept at "covering his tracks," but eventually things caught up with him.

Brad's troubles were not new. When he was a teenager his

parents had frequently bailed him out of trouble, mostly for petty offenses such as vandalism and fighting, but also for sexually assaulting a twelve-year-old female cousin and for pawning a piece of his mother's jewelry that had been in the family for generations. School had presented no problems for him, he said. "I was bright enough to get through college without studying very hard. Some of my classes were pretty large and I sometimes got someone else to take my place during exams." While in law school he was caught with drugs in his possession, but he managed to avoid being charged by claiming that they belonged to someone else.

After serving eighteen months for his last offense, Brad was granted parole. However, two months later he was picked up for attempting to cross the border in his mother's car (taken without her permission), and his parole was revoked.

In our interviews, Brad came across as very pleasant and convincing. As for his victims, he said that nobody was really hurt: "The Law Society has a fund to cover these things. I've more than paid the price by being locked up." The fact is, his law partners and his family suffered large losses because of his actions.

GIVEN THEIR PERSONALITY, it comes as no surprise that psychopaths make good imposters. They have no hesitation in forging and brazenly using impressive credentials to adopt, chameleonlike, professional roles that give them prestige and power. When things begin to fall apart, as they usually do, they simply pack up and move on.

In most cases they select professions in which the requisite skills are easy to fake, the jargon is easy to learn, and the credentials are unlikely to be thoroughly checked. If the profession also places a high premium on the ability to persuade or manipulate others, or to "lay on the hands," so much the better. Thus, psychopaths find it easy to pose as financial consultants, ministers, counselors, and psychologists. But some of their other poses are much more difficult to pull off.

There are psychopaths who sometimes pose as medical doctors, and they may diagnose, dispense drugs, and even perform surgery. That they frequently endanger the health or lives of their patients does not bother them in the least. Ten years ago in Vancouver there was a man who posed as an orthopedic surgeon. For almost a year he performed operations—most of them simple but a few difficult—lived a lavish, high-profile life-style, and was active in social and charitable functions. When questions began to be asked about his sexual relations with his patients, his medical procedures, and several botched operations, he simply disappeared, leaving behind an embarrassed medical community and a number of physically and emotionally damaged patients. A few years later he turned up in England, where he was arrested and jailed for posing as a psychiatrist. At his trial it was learned that at various times he had posed as a social worker, a police officer, an undercover customs agent, and a psychologist specializing in marital problems. Asked how he had managed to slip into so many roles, he replied, "I read a lot." His sentence was short. He may now be in your community.

Targeting the Vulnerable

The idea that a psychopath could actually hang up a shingle as a lawyer or an investment counselor is not very comforting. But even more unsettling are the coldly calculated violations of power and trust committed by a small number of professionals— doctors, psychiatrists, psychologists, teachers, counselors, child-care workers—whose very job it is to help the vulnerable. In *The Mask of Sanity*, for example, Hervey Cleckley vividly described a psychopathic physician and psychiatrist. He noted that the real difference between them and the psychopaths who end up in jail or in psychiatric hospitals is that they simply manage to keep up a better and more consistent appearance of normality. However, their cloak of respectability is thin and uncomfortable and easily shed, often to the dismay of their unfortunate patients. Most common are the therapists who callously use their positions to take sexual advantage of their patients, leaving them feeling bewildered and betrayed. And if the victims complain, they may be traumatized further by a system primed to believe the therapist: "My patient is clearly disturbed, hungry for affection, and prone to fantasy."

The most frightening use of trust to satisfy one's own needs involves the most vulnerable members of society. The number of children who are sexually abused by parents, other relatives, child-care workers, clergymen, and teachers is truly staggering. The most terrifying of the abusers are psychopaths, who think nothing of inflicting devastating physical and emotional damage on the children in their care. Unlike other abusers, many of whom were themselves abused as children, are psychologically disturbed, and often experience anguish about what they are doing, psychopathic abusers are unmoved—"I just take what's available," said one of our subjects, convicted of sexually assaulting his girlfriend's eight-year-old daughter.

Several months ago I received a call from a psychiatrist in a western state. She commented that more than a few private agencies contracted by the state to treat disturbed and delinquent adolescents had been charged with abusing the clients in their care. Her experience with these agencies led her to suspect that many of the offending personnel were psychopaths who willingly used their positions of power and trust to sexually mistreat their patients. She proposed that the *Psychopathy Checklist* be used to screen the personnel of private agencies that bid for custodial and treatment contracts.

Doing What Comes Naturally

There is certainly no shortage of psychopaths who con people into doing things for them, usually to obtain money, prestige, power, or, when incarcerated, freedom. In a sense, it is difficult to see how they could do otherwise, given a personality that makes them "naturals" for the job. Add those universal door-openers—good looks and the gift of gab—and we have a potent recipe for a life of scams and swindles, as someone like Brad could attest.

Their job is made a lot easier simply because a lot of people are surprisingly gullible, with an unshakable belief in the inherent goodness of man.

A recent newspaper article was headlined CON ARTIST'S LATEST PLOY—TELLING THE TRUTH.[18] It described the exploits of a man who became Man of the Year, president of the Chamber of Commerce (shades of serial killer John Wayne Gacy, whose bid for Jaycee president was interrupted by his first murder conviction), and member of the Republican Executive Committee in the small town where he had resided for ten years. Billing himself as a Berkeley Ph.D. in psychology, he decided to run for a place on the local school board. "That pays $18,000," he later said. "And I thought I could parlay that into the county commission, which is $30,000. Then maybe state rep."

A local reporter decided to check this man's credentials from information the latter had supplied. Except for the place and date of birth, all the data were fictitious. ("Always mix in a little truth," he told the reporter, offering this advice for free.) Not only was the man a complete impostor, as the reporter discovered, but he had a long history of antisocial behavior, fraud, impersonation, and imprisonment, and his only contact with a university involved extension courses he'd taken while serving time in Leavenworth Federal Penitentiary. "Before he was a con man he was a con boy. He was the kind of kid who would steal a Boy Scout uniform in order to hitchhike. He would tell people that he had hit the road to earn a merit badge. Later he joined the army, only to desert after three weeks. Then he masqueraded as a flier in the Royal Air Force. He persuaded people he was a hero. . . . For two decades he dodged across America, a step ahead of the hoodwinked. Along the way he picked up three wives, three divorces, and four children. To this day he has no idea of what happened to any of them."

When found out, this man was unconcerned, and stated that he knew that if he was ever discovered "these trusting people would stand behind me. A good liar is a good judge of people," he added, a remark that probably had more truth in it than everything else he had said put together. His only embarrassment was that it was merely a local reporter who had found him out. Even so, he was able to dismiss the fellow's investigative coup with the offhand comment, "I had an easy cover."

Perhaps most remarkable in this account, although by no means unusual, was the fact that far from decrying this fellow's outrageous program of deception, the local community he had conned so thoroughly rushed to his support. And it was not merely token support they offered. "I assess [his] genuineness, integrity, and devotion to duty to rank right alongside of President Abraham Lincoln," wrote the Republican party chairman. Presumably, he was more swayed by the impostor's words than by his deeds. Or perhaps he, and the rest of the community, could not come to grips with the fact that they had been taken in. As one commentator put it, "There is no crime in the cynical American calendar more humiliating than to be a sucker."[19]

This of course makes life a lot easier for the con artist and the fraud. Our impostor saw the doors opening to him right away and began to make new plans to enter the political arena. "Name recognition is so important to a politician, and more people know my name than before," he said. "I can run with this for years." Most of us would be devastated and humiliated by public exposure as a liar and a cheat, but not the psychopath. He or she can still look the community straight in the eye and give impassioned assurances, on their "word of honor."

IN A CASE that struck uncomfortably close to home, I was invited to speak about my research on psychopaths at a conference on crime in California, and was to receive an honorarium of five hundred dollars plus expenses. Six months after the conference, I still had not been paid, so I made inquiries and learned that the organizer had been arrested at a government meeting in Washington and charged with several counts of fraud, forgery, and theft. It turned out that he had a long criminal record, had been diagnosed by several psychiatrists as a "classic psychopath," and had forged the documents and letters of reference used to obtain his job. Needless to say, I was not the only speaker who had not been paid. To top things off, shortly after my talk he sent me a copy—complete with editorial comments—of an article on the diagnosis of psychopathy. Following his arrest, he was let out on bail and has since disappeared.

Ironically, I had spent quite a bit of time with this man, at a luncheon held just before my talk and later in a bar. I detected nothing unusual or suspicious about him; my antenna failed to twitch in his presence. Would I have lent him money? Possibly. I do recall insisting that I pick up the bar tab. He wasn't wearing a bell around his neck!

Subcriminal Psychopaths

Many psychopaths wind up in prisons or other correctional facilities time and again. The characteristic pattern is a lifelong bouncing from one job or another into jail and then back onto the streets, into and out of prison, perhaps into a mental health facility and quickly out, once the staff realizes they have on their hands a patient who is bound to make trouble and disrupt the institutional routine. The net effect in the typical case is that of a Ping Pong ball out of control.

However, many psychopaths never go to prison or any other facility. They appear to function reasonably well—as lawyers, doctors, psychiatrists, academics, mercenaries, police officers, cult leaders, military personnel, businesspeople, writers, artists, entertainers, and so forth—without breaking the law, or at least without being caught and convicted. These individuals are every bit as egocentric, callous, and manipulative as the average criminal psychopath; however, their intelligence, family background, social skills, and circumstances permit them to construct a facade of normalcy and to get what they want with relative impunity.

Some commentators refer to them as "successful psychopaths." Others argue that individuals of this sort benefit society. Just as they are able to ignore society's rules, the argument goes, intelligent psychopaths are able to transcend the bounds of conventional thought, providing a creative spark for the arts, the theater, design, and so on. Whatever the merits of this argument, they are more than offset—in my view—by the broken hearts, shattered careers, and used-up people left in their wake as they cut a zigzag route through society, driven by a remorseless need to "express themselves."

Rather than refer to these individuals as successful psychopaths—after all, their success is often illusory and always at someone else's expense—I prefer to call them *subcriminal* psychopaths. Their conduct, although technically not illegal, typically violates conventional ethical standards, hovering just on the shady side of the law. Unlike people who consciously adopt a ruthless, greedy, and apparently unscrupulous strategy in their business dealings but who are reasonably honest and empathetic in other areas of their lives, subcriminal psychopaths exhibit much the same behaviors and attitudes in *all* areas of their lives. If they lie and cheat on the job—and get away with it or are even admired for it—they will lie and cheat in other areas of their lives.

> TWO BUSINESSMEN ARE walking together, each carrying a briefcase. "We're only *morally* bankrupt," says one. "Thank God," says the other.
> —From a cartoon by Bill Lee in *Omni*,
> March 1991, p. 84

I am certain that if the families and friends of such individuals were willing to discuss their experiences without fear of retribution, we would uncover a rat's nest of emotional abuse, philandering, double-dealing, and generally shoddy behavior. These rat's nests are sometimes made public in dramatic fashion. Think of the many high-profile cases in which a "pillar of the community" commits a serious crime—say, murder or rape—and in the process of investigations by the police and news media the perpetrator's dark side is revealed. Many such cases are vividly portrayed in books and movies, and the shocked—and titillated—public asks, "Where did they go wrong?" and, "What made them do it?"

The answer, in most cases, is that the culprit didn't just suddenly "go wrong." Individuals who frequent the shady side of the law stand a good chance of slipping over the edge. In such cases, the crime is simply a natural consequence of a deviant personality structure that has always been present but that, because of good luck, social skills, cover-ups, a fearful family, or friends and associates who conveniently refused to see what was going on, had not previously resulted in a criminal act that came to the attention of the justice system.

Think, for example, of John Gacy (*Buried Dreams*), Jeffrey Mac-

Donald (*Fatal Vision*), Ted Bundy (*The Stranger Beside Me*), Diane Downs (*Small Sacrifices*), Kevin Coe (*Son*), Angelo Buono and Kenneth Bianchi (*Two of a Kind: The Hillside Stranglers*), David Brown (*Love, Lies and Murder*), and Kenneth Taylor (*In the Name of the Child*), to name but a few of the more sensational cases that have been described in books and have become well known.

We now diagnose most of these people as psychopaths, but the crucial point here is that their disorder and its behavior did not suddenly appear full-blown out of nowhere. *They were the same people before they were caught as they were afterward.* They are psychopaths now and they were psychopaths before.

This is a disturbing thought, because it suggests that the cases that come to the public's attention represent only the tip of a very large iceberg.

The rest of the iceberg is to be found nearly everywhere—in business, the home, the professions, the military, the arts, the entertainment industry, the news media, academe, and the blue-collar world. Millions of men, women, and children daily suffer terror, anxiety, pain, and humiliation at the hands of the psychopaths in their lives.

Tragically, these victims often cannot get other people to understand what they are going through. Psychopaths are very good at putting on a good impression when it suits them, and they often paint their victims as the real culprits. As one woman—the third wife of a forty-year-old high school teacher—recently told me: "For five years he cheated on me, kept me living in fear, and forged checks on my personal bank account. But everyone, including my doctor and lawyer and my friends, blamed *me* for the problem. He had them so convinced that he was a great guy and that I was going mad, I began to believe it myself. Even when he cleaned out my bank account and ran off with a seventeen-year-old student, a lot of people couldn't believe it, and some wanted to know what *I* had done to make him act so strangely."

IN THE APRIL 1, 1990 edition of *The New York Times* Daniel Goleman wrote about Robert Hogan's work on managers and executives who display the "dark side of charisma." Hogan, a psychologist at the Tulsa Institute of Behavioral Sciences, described "flawed managers, whose glittering image masks a dark destructive side" and who "act as if the normal rules don't apply to them. But they climb the corporate ladder quickly; they're outstanding at self-promotion," he said. "While they muster a charming performance, it's a snake's charm, like J.R. Ewing on *Dallas.*" Referring to psychologist Harry Levinson's work on healthy and unhealthy narcissism in managers, Hogan noted that unhealthy narcissists have an almost grandiose sense of certainty and a disdain for subordinates. "They are particularly good at ingratiating themselves with their seniors but brutalize their juniors," he is quoted as saying.

A Corporate Psychopath

The following case study was kindly provided by Paul Babiak, an industrial/organizational psychologist in New York:

Dave is in his midthirties. He has a B.A. from a state college, is married for the third time, and has four children. He was brought to Babiak's attention as a "problem employee" by his boss during an organizational study of a major corporation in Colorado. He had done extremely well on interviews, so his boss was surprised when things started to go wrong.

Dave's boss discovered that the first major report he produced included large amounts of plagiarized material. When confronted, Dave brushed aside the concern, commenting that he considered it a poor use of his time and talents to "reinvent the wheel." He frequently "forgot" to work on certain uninteresting projects and on at least one occassion sent his boss a memo saying that he was unwilling to take on additional assignments.

Babiak interviewed other employees in the department and began to sense that Dave was the source of most of the department's conflicts. Co-workers gave him numerous examples of Dave's disruptive behavior. For example, he was told that shortly after joining the department Dave got into a yelling match with his boss's secretary, then stormed into his boss's office and demanded that she be fired because she had dared to refuse to come in on Saturday (with no notice). *Her* version of the incident was somewhat different: Dave had been rude and condescending to her and was upset that she would not drop everything to cater to his requests. Dave was frequently unprepared and late for staff meetings. When he did show up he could be counted on to deliver a verbal tirade. When his boss asked him to control his outbursts, Dave responded that in his opinion fighting and aggression were necessary forces and that people needed them to advance in life. His boss commented that he never seemed to learn from the feedback he received, never acknowledged that he had done anything wrong, and always acted surprised when given feedback, insisting that he had never been told that he had done anything wrong before.

Dave's co-workers were consistent in their descriptions—they found him rude, selfish, immature, self-centered, unreliable, and irresponsible. Virtually all reported that they initially liked him but over time grew to distrust him, and they said that they knew the stories he used to gain their cooperation were lies. Still, they went along with him because they didn't want to "call him" on his fabrications. Some employees who claimed to be "wise to him" said that virtually everything he said was a lie and his promises were never to be believed.

During his meeting with Babiak, Dave described himself as a hard worker, a strong leader, a "team builder," honest, intelligent, the guy responsible for really "making" the department. In fact, he suggested that his boss leave the company and he take over. (His boss said that Dave had made the same suggestion to him directly.) He also commented that his *real* boss was the president of the corporation. He came across as quite egotistical, but not necessarily concerned about how others felt about him. His attitudes and choice of words left the impression that people were mere objects to him.

In checking Dave's credentials several discrepancies turned up. For example, his major field of study differed from resumé to application form. A third document, a letter, listed still a third field of study. Babiak brought these to the attention of Dave's boss (who had never noticed), and he sent a memo to Dave asking him for an explanation. Dave sent the boss's memo back with the erroneous degree crossed off and a fourth variation written in! When confronted, he grew defiant and then brushed off the concern with a comment that there was nothing wrong in claiming different majors for different purposes, since he'd taken courses in all the subjects he'd mentioned.

Armed with evidence of improprieties in Dave's expense account, Dave's boss went to *his* boss with complaints about Dave, only to learn that Dave had been complaining about *him* from the start. After hearing the "other side" of a lot of stories, the executive suggested a test of Dave's integrity. They agreed on some information to be conveyed to Dave by his boss the next morning. This meeting took place as planned and Dave subsequently called the higher-level executive for a private meeting. At this meeting, he relayed the "information" about his boss, all of it distorted. This convinced the executive that Dave was a liar and was trying to undermine his boss. Surprisingly, however, subsequent action against Dave was blocked by several members of upper management.

What interested Babiak most about this case was the fact that while those closest to him were convinced of Dave's manipulations, irresponsibility, and lack of integrity, those higher up in the organization had been convinced—by Dave—of his management talent and potential. Despite clear evidence of dishonesty, they were still "charmed" by him. His ranting and raving behavior were excused as part of his creative, almost artistic, bent, while his aggression and backbiting were seen by those people as "ambition." Dave's ability to manage the discrepant views of these two groups of people led Babiak to seek a more systematic evaluation of his personality.

Not surprisingly, Dave received a high score on the *Psychopathy Checklist*. His personality and behaviors made him different from the typical "problem employee" seen in organizations.

Dave has actually been quite successful from an organizational point of view; he's had two promotions in two years, received regular salary increases (despite a negative performance evaluation by his boss), and has been included in a corporate succession plan as a high-potential employee. Babiak also sees him as successful from a psychological point of view, owing to his ability to manipulate upper management into believing his view of things for more than two years. This is especially notable when we realize that his peers, subordinates, and immediate supervisor saw him exhibiting behaviors and traits that researchers normally ascribe to psychopaths.

Rich Feeding Grounds

There is no shortage of opportunities for white-collar psychopaths who think big. The business pages of every major newspaper routinely contain reports of investigations into shady money-making schemes and deals concocted and operated by con artists and scam masters. These reports cover only a small number of the thousands of lucrative opportunities that exist for a fast-talking psychopath with a head for numbers and the social skills to move easily in financial circles. For these individuals, the potential for profit is so enormous, the rules so flexible, and the watchdogs so sleepy that they must feel they have found paradise. A few recent examples, one modest and the others far less so, illustrate the scope of the watering holes available to, and certainly used by, enterprising psychopaths:

• An article in *Forbes* headed SCAM CAPITAL OF THE WORLD described the Vancouver Stock Exchange as "infested with crooked promoters, sons of crooked promoters and sons of friends of crooked promoters." Local newspapers continually report a litany of scams, swindles, phony stock promotions, and blatant hype designed to boost share prices on the Exchange. Penalties for being caught are often laughable, and they certainly do little to dampen the wild and voracious scheming. If I were unable to study psychopaths in prison, my next choice would very likely be a place like the Vancouver Stock Exchange.

• In the late 1980s, the lid blew off a decade's worth of rotten investments, phony promises, fraudulent business practices, and voracious greed in the United States savings and loan (S & L) business, which President Reagan had deregulated in the early 1980s. Without the pressure to conform to the rules under strict governmental oversight, certain S & L personnel began to take freedoms with their depositors' money that led, in a gradually building avalanche of debt, to a financial disaster of unprecedented proportions. At the time of this writing, the projected cost to U.S. taxpayers of what has become known as the S & L bail-out approaches $1 *trillion*—more than the entire cost of the Vietnam War.

• Incredible at it seems, even the S & L scandals have been topped by recent revelations of a worldwide network of unbelievable greed and corruption. "Nothing in the history of modern financial scandals rivals the unfolding saga of the bank of Credit and Commerce International, the $20 billion rogue empire that regulators in 62 countries shut down. . . . in a stunning global sweep. Never has a scandal involved so much money, so many nations, and so many prominent people. . . . Superlatives are quickly exhausted: it is the largest corporate criminal enterprise ever. . . . the most pervasive money-laundering operation and financial supermarket ever created."[20]

AT THIS WRITING, the mysterious death of publishing czar Robert Maxwell has opened an enormous can of worms. Maxwell's business empire collapsed amid charges that hundreds of millions of dollars were illegally siphoned off. The case is relevant here as a good example of how a carefully managed public persona can conceal dark deeds and a black heart.

Although it was widely known that he was a crook and a charlatan who was adept at moving money from one company to another, most of those who knew him, including journalists, managed to keep remarkably silent. Maxwell had a great deal of power and was able to intimidate his critics. He also benefited from the "unscrupulousness of greed" and an establishment that turns a blind eye toward "unconvicted money-making crooks." (Quotes are from an article by Peter Jenkins, "Captain Bob Revealed: A Crook and a Conspiracy of Silence." *Independent News Service*, December 7, 1991.)

They've Got What it Takes

It is not difficult to see why psychopaths are so attracted to and so successful at white-collar crime. First, lots of juicy opportunities present themselves. As one of our subjects, convicted of selling forged corporate bonds, put it, "I wouldn't be in prison if there weren't so many cookie jars just begging me to put my hand in." His cookie jars were pension funds, boiler-room stock promotions, charity fund-raising drives, and shared-vacation condo schemes, only a few of the many well-furnished niches that allow those of his ilk to operate unobtrusively.

Second, psychopaths have what it takes to defraud and bilk others: They are fast-talking, charming, self-assured, at ease in social situations, cool under pressure, unfazed by the possibility of being found out, and totally ruthless. And even when exposed, they can carry on as if nothing has happened, often leaving their accusers bewildered and uncertain about their own positions.

Finally, white-collar crime is lucrative, the chances of getting caught are minimal, and the penalties are often trivial. Think of the insider traders, junk-bond kings, and S & L sharks whose financial depredations were so spectacularly rewarding—even when they were caught. In many cases, the rules of the game for greed and fraud carried out on a grand scale are not the same as they are for ordinary crime. Often, the players in the former form a loosely structured network to protect their mutual interests: They come from the same social strata and the same schools, belong to the same clubs, and may even be instrumental in setting up the rules in the first place. A bank robber may be sentenced to twenty years in prison, whereas a lawyer, businessperson, or politician who defrauds the public out of millions of dollars may receive a fine or a suspended sentence, usually after a trial marked by long delays, adjournments, and obscure legal maneuvers. We condemn and shun the bank robber but ask the embezzler to help us invest our money or join our tennis club.

THE LAWYER FOR one of the individuals (Mr. X) involved in recent insider-trading scandals traveled to Vancouver to enlist my aid in defending his client, who had been "fingered" by another player in the game (Mr. Y). The lawyer proposed that I use the *Psychopathy Checklist* to determine if the man who had named his client was a psychopath, and, saying that "money is no object," suggested that I might want to interview Mr. Y's friends, business associates, former classmates, and neighbors. He also said that I could be set up in a beach house near the one Mr. Y frequently used, and that all I had to do was to get to know him well enough to complete the checklist on him. When I inquired why it would be useful for him to know whether Mr. Y was a psychopath, the attorney replied that it could be crucial to his case because, as everyone knows, psychopaths are notoriously deceitful, unreliable, and eager to save their own skin at any cost. If Mr. Y could be diagnosed as a psychopath, his testimony might be discredited and the lawyer would have a better chance of working out a reasonable plea bargain with the state. Although I might have become very wealthy—"money is no object"—I declined the offer.

Unfortunately, many people do not consider white-collar crime as serious as crimes aimed directly at people, such as robbery or rape. In the case described at the beginning of this chapter, John Grambling made the following plea to the judge who was about to sentence him:

> I have been sitting in jail now for two months and have experienced living in a cell with a poor ignorant illegal alien, a career criminal, a drug user and smuggler, and a killer. I have reached rock bottom in my emotions and esteem by having to spend time with this element of society, and yet I am here and by some logic should be considered similar to them. I can tell you without hesitation I am *not* at all similar. I don't look the same, talk the same, act the same, or feel the same.[21]

The judge in the case commented that, although he disagreed with Grambling, "in practice there is a difference between a crime against a person and a crime against property. . . . between someone who rapes you, or threatens to rape you, or threatens to kill or threatens to maim, and someone who may cause as much damage with a fountain pen."[22] The prosecutor noted, "The federal prisons for the wealthy and privileged . . . have tasty food, jogging tracks, first-run movies, and libraries. . . . The federal prisons for the rich and privileged are a national disgrace."[23]

These messages are not lost on the psychopath who has a yen for the high life.

Chapter 8

Words from
an Overcoat Pocket

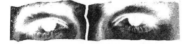

A word is not the same with one writer as with another.
One tears it from his guts. The other pulls it out of his
overcoat pocket.
      —Charles Peguy, "The Honest People,"
      Basic Verities (1943), tr. Ann and Julian Green

One question runs like a refrain through the stories told
by the victims of psychopaths: *"How* could I have been so stupid? How could I have fallen for that incredible line of baloney?"

And when victims aren't asking themselves, somebody else
is sure to pose the question. "How on earth could you have
been taken in to that extent?" The characteristic answer: "You
had to be there. It seemed reasonable, plausible at the time."
The clear—and largely valid—implication is that *had* we been
there we too might have been sucked in.

Some people are simply too trusting and gullible for their own
good—ready targets for any smooth talker who comes along.
But what about the rest of us? The sad fact is that we are all
vulnerable. Few people are such sophisticated and perceptive
judges of human nature that they cannot be taken in by the
machinations of a skilled and determined psychopath. Even
those who study them are not immune; as I've indicated in

previous chapters, my students and I are sometimes conned, even when aware that we're dealing with a probable psychopath.

Of course, pathological lying and manipulation are not restricted to psychopaths. What makes psychopaths different from all others is the remarkable ease with which they lie, the pervasiveness of their deception, and the callousness with which they carry it out.

But there is something else about the speech of psychopaths that is equally puzzling: their frequent use of contradictory and logically inconsistent statements that usually escape detection. Recent research on the language of psychopaths provides us with some important clues to this puzzle, as well as to the uncanny ability psychopaths have to move words—and people—around so easily. But first, here are some examples to illustrate the point, the first three from offenders who scored high on the *Psychopathy Checklist.*

- When asked if he had ever committed a violent offense, a man serving time for theft answered, "No, but I once had to kill someone."

- A woman with a staggering record of fraud, deceit, lies, and broken promises concluded a letter to the parole board with, "I've let a lot of people down. . . . One is only as good as her reputation and name. My word is as good as gold."

- A man serving a term for armed robbery replied to the testimony of an eyewitness, "He's lying. I wasn't there. I should have blown his fucking head off."

- A tabloid television program showed a classic con man who shamelessly swindled elderly women.[1] When the interviewer asked, "Where do you draw the line between right and wrong?" he replied, "I have some morals, whether you believe it or not, I have some morals." To the interviewer's question, "And where do you draw the line?" he replied, "That's a good question. I'm not trying to hedge, but that's a good question." When asked, "Did

125

you actually carry around in your briefcase blank power-of-attorney forms?" his reply was, "No, I didn't carry them around, but I had them in my briefcase, yes."

- When Ted Bundy was asked what cocaine did to him he replied, "Cocaine? I've never used it. . . . I've never tried cocaine. I think I might have tried it once and got nothing out of it. Just snorted a little bit. And I just don't mess with it. It's too expensive. And I suppose if I was on the streets and had enough of it, I might get into it. But I'm strictly a marijuana man. All I do is . . . I *love* to smoke a reefer. And Valiums. And of course alcohol."[2]

Think about this for a moment—not only lies but several contradictory statements in the same breath. Very perplexing. It is as if psychopaths sometimes have difficulty in monitoring their own speech, and they let loose with a convoluted barrage of poorly connected words and thoughts.

Psychopaths also sometimes put words together in strange ways. For example, consider the following exchange between a journalist and psychopathic serial killer, Clifford Olson. "And then I had *annual* sex with her." "Once a year?" "No. Annual. From behind." "Oh. But she was dead!" "No, no. She was just *unconscientious*." About his many experiences, Olson said, "I've got enough *antidotes* to fill five or six books—enough for a *trilogy*." He was determined not to be an *"escape goat"* no matter what the *"migrating* facts."[3] [emphasis mine]

Of course, words don't simply pop out of our mouths of their own accord. They are the end products of very complicated mental activity. This raises the interesting possibility that, like much of their behavior, the mental processes of psychopaths are poorly regulated and not bound by conventional rules. This issue is discussed in the following sections, which outline evidence that psychopaths differ from others in the way their brains are organized and in the connections between words and emotion. In the next chapter I take up the related issue of why the listener often fails to notice the psychopath's verbal quirks.

A CONVICTED SERIAL killer, Elmer Wayne Henley, now asking for parole, says that he was the victim of an older serial killer he worked with, and that he would not have done anything wrong on his own. Together, they killed at least twenty-seven young men and boys. "I'm passive," he offered. "I don't want to be no psychopath, I don't want to be no killer. I just want to be decent people."

Consider the following exchange between the interviewer and Henley. The interviewer says, "You make it out that you're the victim of a serial killer, but if you look at the record you're a serial killer." Henley replies, "I'm not." "You're not a serial killer?" the interviewer asks in disbelief, to which Henley replies, "I'm not a serial killer." The interviewer then says, "You're saying you're not a serial killer now, but you've serially killed." Henley replies, with some exasperation and condescension, "Well, yeah, that's semantics."

—From the May 8, 1991, episode of *48 Hours*

Who's in Charge?

In most people the two sides of the brain have different, specialized functions. The left cerebral hemisphere is skilled at processing information analytically and sequentially, and it plays a crucial role in the understanding and use of language. The right hemisphere processes information simultaneously, as a whole; it plays an important role in the perception of spatial relations, imagery, emotional experience, and the processing of music.

Nature probably "arranged" for each side of the brain to have different functions for the sake of efficiency.[4] For example, it is clearly more effective for all the complex mental operations required to use and understand language to take place in one side of the brain than if they were distributed over both sides. In the latter case, information would have to be sent back and forth between the two hemispheres, which would slow down the processing rate and increase the chances of error.

Further, *some* part of the brain has to have primary control over the task; if the two sides of the brain were competing for this control, the conflict would reduce the efficiency of processing. Some forms of dyslexia and stuttering, for example, are associated with just such a condition: Language centers are bilateral—located in *both* hemispheres. Competition between the two hemispheres makes for a variety of difficulties in the understanding and production of language.

New experimental evidence suggests that bilateral language processes are also characteristic of psychopathy.[5] This leads me to speculate that part of the tendency for psychopaths to make contradictory statements is related to an inefficient "line of authority"—each hemisphere tries to run the show, with the result that speech is poorly integrated and monitored.

Of course, others with bilateral language—some stutterers, dyslexics, and left-handers—do not lie and contradict themselves the way psychopaths do. Clearly, something else must be involved.

Hollow Words

Most people who have had extensive experience with psychopaths have an intuitive sense of what that difference might be. "He was always telling me how much he loved me, and at first I believed him, even after I caught him fooling around with my sister," said the estranged wife of one of our psychopathic subjects. "It took me a long time to realize that he didn't care for me at all. Every time he beat up on me he would say, 'I'm really sorry, pigeon. You know I love you.' Right out of a cheap movie!"

This would come as no surprise to clinicians, long aware that psychopaths seem to know the dictionary meanings of words but fail to comprehend or appreciate their *emotional* value or significance. Consider the following quotes from the clinical literature on psychopathy:

- "He knows the words but not the music."[6]

- "Ideas of mutuality of sharing and understanding are beyond his understanding in an emotional sense; he knows only the book meaning of words."[7]

- "[He] exhibits a facility with words that mean little to him, form without substance. . . . His seemingly good judgment and social sense are only word deep."[8]

These clinical observations get right to the heart of the mystery of psychopathy: language that is two-dimensional, lacking in emotional depth.

A simple analogy here will help. The psychopath is like a color-blind person who sees the world in shades of gray but who has learned how to function in a colored world. He has learned that the light signal for "stop" is at the top of the traffic signal. When the color-blind person tells you he stopped at the *red* light, he really means he stopped at the *top* light. He has difficulty in discussing the color of things but may have learned all sorts of ways to compensate for this problem, and in some cases even those who know him well may not know that he cannot see colors.

Like the color-blind person, the psychopath lacks an important element of experience—in this case, emotional experience—but may have learned the words that others use to describe or mimic experiences that he cannot really understand. As Cleckley put it, "He can learn to use ordinary words . . . [and] will also learn to reproduce appropriately all the pantomime of feeling . . . but the feeling itself does not come to pass."[9]

Recent laboratory research provides convincing support for these clinical observations. This research is based on evidence that, for normal people, neutral words generally convey less information than do emotional words: A word such as PAPER has dictionary meaning, whereas a word such as DEATH has dictionary meaning *plus* emotional meaning and unpleasant connotations. Emotional words have more "punch" than do other words.

Picture yourself sitting before a computer screen on which groups of letters are flashed for a fraction of a second. Electrodes for recording brain responses have been attached to your scalp and connected to an EEG machine, which draws a graph of the electrical activity of the brain. Some of the groups of letters flashed on the screen form common words found in the dictionary; other strings form no words, only nonsense syllables. For example, TREE forms a word but RETE does not. Your task is to push a button as quickly as possible whenever you have decided that a true *word* appeared on the screen. The computer measures the time it takes you to make your decision; it also analyzes your brain responses during the task.

You will probably respond more quickly to an emotional word than to a neutral one. For example, you—and most other people—would push the button more quickly at the word DEATH than at the word PAPER. The emotional content of a word seems to give a sort of "turbo-boost" to the decision-making process. At the same time, the emotional words evoke *larger* brain responses than do neutral words, a reflection of the relatively large amount of information contained in the emotional words.

A PSYCHOPATHIC KILLER, asked by a female interviewer to explain the motivations for his crimes, instead launched into a graphic description of several particularly brutal murders and mutilations for which he had been imprisoned. His account was animated but dispassionate, as if he were describing a baseball game. At first the interviewer tried to appear nonjudgmental and to show only professional interest in the account. However, when her facial expression finally betrayed her revulsion he stopped in midsentence and said, "Yeah, I guess it was pretty bad. I really feel rotten. I must have been temporarily insane."

Like most people, psychopaths sometimes say and do things solely to impress or shock. However, because of their sparse emotional life they don't intuitively realize the impact on others of what they say. They use their listeners' reactions as "cue cards" to tell them how they are *supposed* to feel in the situation.

When we used this laboratory task with prison inmates, the nonpsychopaths showed the normal pattern of responses—quicker decisions and larger brain responses to emotional than to neutral words—but the psychopaths did not: *They responded to emotional words as if they were neutral words.*[10] This dramatic finding provided strong support for the argument that words do not have the same emotional or affective coloring for psychopaths as they do for other people. Some of our more recent research provides additional support for this thesis, confirming that, for whatever reason, psychopaths lack some of the "feelable" components of language.[11]

This deficiency has fascinating implications, especially when considered in the context of psychopaths' social interactions—manipulative deceit uninhibited by empathy or conscience. For most of us, language has the capacity to elicit powerful emotional feelings. For example, the word *cancer* evokes not only a clinical description of a disease and its symptoms but a sense of fear, apprehension, or concern, and perhaps disturbing mental images of what it might be like to have it. But to the psychopath, a word is just a word.

Brain-imaging technology offers the prospect of gaining exciting new insights into the emotional life of psychopaths. In a collaborative research project at the Mt. Sinai and Bronx VA Medical Centers in New York, led by psychiatrist Joanne Intrator, we recently began to obtain brain-images from psychopathic and normal individuals while they performed a variety of tasks. Our preliminary findings from a pilot project (presented at the annual meetings of the Society for Biological Psychiatry and the American Psychiatric Association in San Francisco, May, 1993), suggest that psychopaths may not use the same areas of the brain that normal individuals do when they process emotional words. If these results can be replicated and extended to other forms of emotional information, they would suggest that psychopaths differ from others either in the strategies they use to process emotional material or in the way their brain processes are organized. In either case, we would be considerably closer than we are now to understanding the mystery of the psychopath.

In a book explaining her side of the shooting of her three children, Diane Downs described her causal relationships with a score of men as loveless, motivated only by sex.[12] In letters sent to Robert Bertaluccini ("Bert"), a fellow letter carrier, she wrote of her "promises of undying love, endless devotion and oaths that no one else on earth would ever touch me. It was the game I played with men. And I played it best with Bert." [p. 144] After shooting her children she had an affair with Jason Redding, and wrote, "But Bert was in the past, and Jason was in the present. True, I was writing letters to Bert telling him how much I loved him, that he was the only man on earth for me. . . . When he began to refuse the letters, I started saving them in a notebook, making an entry each night, most of them a paragraph or two, a page at most. The entries were the same, just with different wording: 'I love you Bert, why aren't you here, I need you, you're the only man for me.' . . . I mixed a drink and wrote my hollow words of love to Bert as I sank into a hot bubble bath. . . . I thought about Bert. . . . Minutes later Jason knocked at the door, and as I flew down the stairs to meet him, my thoughts of Bert flew as well." [pp. 36–37] Diane's "hollow words of love" were a source of pride to her, as if their use was entirely intentional, designed for a particular purpose. However, like all psychopaths, *her words of love could not be anything but hollow,* for she lacks the capacity to impart real feeling to them.

Earlier I discussed the role of "inner speech" in the development and operation of conscience. It is the *emotionally charged* thoughts, images, and internal dialogue that give the "bite" to conscience, account for its powerful control over behavior, and generate guilt and remorse for transgressions. This is something that psychopaths cannot understand. For them, conscience is little more than an intellectual awareness of rules others make up—empty words. The feelings needed to give clout to these rules are missing. The question is, why?

CANADA's MOST NOTORIOUS and reviled criminal is Clifford Olson, a serial murderer sentenced in January 1982 to life imprisonment for the torture and killing of eleven boys and girls. These crimes were the latest and most despicable in a string of antisocial and criminal acts extending back to his early childhood. Although some psychopaths are not violent and few are as brutal as he, Olson is the prototypical psychopath.

Consider the following quotations from a newspaper article written around the time of his trial: "He was a braggart and a bully, a liar and a thief. He was a violent man with a hairtrigger temper. But he could also be charming and smooth-tongued when trying to impress people ... Olson was a compulsive talker ... He's a real smooth talker, he has the gift of gab ... He was always telling whoppers ... The man was just an out-and-out liar ... He always wanted to test you to the limits. He wanted to see how far he could go before you had to step on him ... He was a manipulator ... Olson was a blabbermouth ... We learned after a while not to believe anything he said because he told so many lies." [Farrow, 1982] A reporter who talked with Olson said, "He talked fast, staccato ... He jumped from topic to topic. He sounded glib, slick, like a con trying to prove he's tough and important." [Ouston, 1982]

These reports by people who knew him are important, for they give us a clue to why he was able to get his young, trusting victims alone with him. They may also help to explain the Crown's decision to pay him $100,000 to tell them where he hid the bodies of seven of the eleven young people he had killed. Not surprisingly, public outrage greeted disclosure of the payment. Some typical headlines were: KILLER WAS PAID TO LOCATE BODIES; MONEY-FOR-GRAVES PAYMENT TO CHILD KILLER GREETED WITH DISGUST.

In the years since his imprisonment Olson has continued to bring grief to the families of his victims by sending them letters with comments about the murders of their children. He has never shown any guilt or remorse for his depredations; on the contrary, he continually complains about his treatment by the press, the prison system, and society. During his trial he preened and postured whenever a camera was present, apparently considering himself an important celebrity rather than a man who had committed a series of atrocities. On January 15, 1983, the *Vancouver Sun* reported, "Mass killer Clifford Olson has written to the *Sun* newsroom to say he does not approve of the picture of him we have been using ... and will shortly be sending us newer, more attractive pictures of himself." [Quotes are from articles by R. Ouston, *Vancouver Sun*, January 15, 1982, and M. Farrow, *Vancouver Sun*, January 14, 1982]

At this writing Olson has written to several criminology departments in Canada offering to help them establish a course devoted to studying him.

Below the Emotional Poverty Line

If the language of psychopaths is bilateral—controlled by both sides of the brain—it is possible that other brain processes normally controlled by one hemisphere are also under bilateral control. Indeed, although in most people the right side of the brain plays a central role in emotion, recent laboratory evidence indicates that in psychopaths *neither* side of the brain is proficient in the processes of emotion.[13] Why this is so is still a mystery. But an intriguing implication is that the brain processes that control the psychopath's emotions are divided and unfocused, resulting in a shallow and colorless emotional life.

Ted Bundy may have been indignant when someone referred to him as an emotional robot with nothing inside. "Boy, how far off can he be!" said Bundy. "If they think I have no emotional life, they're wrong. Absolutely wrong. It's a very real one and a full one."[14] However, it is abundantly clear from his other comments and the shallow explanations for his murderous behavior that the description is apt. Like all psychopaths, Bundy had only a vague comprehension of the extent of his emotional poverty.

Many people are attracted to pop-psych movements that emphasize a search for self-understanding—"getting in touch with your feelings." For psychopaths, the exercise—like the search for the Holy Grail—is doomed to failure. In the final analysis, their self-image is defined more by possessions and other visible signs of success and power than by love, insight, and compassion, which are abstractions and have little inherent meaning for them.

134

Watch Their Hands

Watch the way someone talking to you moves his or her hands: Do they move infrequently or do they fly all over the place? Do the hand gestures help you to understand what is being said? Some do, for they provide visual enhancement to the speaker's words—for example, moving the hands wide apart while saying, "It was a really *big* fish," or tracing out the shape of a person being described.[15]

However, most language-related hand gestures convey no information or meaning to the listener. "Empty" hand gestures called *beats* are small, rapid hand movements that occur only during speech or pauses in speech but are not part of the "story line." Like other gestures and body movements, they are often part of the "show" the speaker puts on (I'll have more to say about this in the following chapter) or a reflection of a culturally based style of communication. But beats occur for other reasons as well. For example, many people make these hand gestures while talking on the telephone. The listener can't see these gestures, so why does the speaker make them?

The answer may be related to evidence that the brain centers that control speech also control the hand gestures made during speech. In some unknown way—perhaps by increasing overall activity in these centers—beats seem to facilitate speech: They help us to put our thoughts and feelings into words. If this sounds strange, watch the frantic hand movements someone makes the next time he or she has trouble finding a word. Or, make a point of *not* using your hands when you speak; is there an increase in the number of hesitations, pauses, and stumbles in your speech? If you speak two languages, you will probably make a lot more beat gestures when speaking in your second language than when speaking in your native tongue. In some cases, a high rate of beat gestures appears to reflect difficulty in converting thoughts and feelings into speech.

Beats may also tell us something about the size of the "thought units," or mental packages, that underlie speech. A thought unit can vary from something small, simple, and isolated—a single idea or word, a phrase, a sentence—to something larger and more complex—groups of ideas, sentences, or complete story lines. The ideas, words, phrases, and sentences that comprise large thought units are likely to be well integrated, tied together in some meaningful, consistent, or logical fashion to form a script. Beats appear to "mark off" these thought units: The greater the number of beats, the smaller the units.

Recent evidence suggests that psychopaths use more beats than do normal people, particularly when they talk about things generally considered *emotional*—for example, describing the way they feel about family members or other "loved ones."[16] We might infer two things from this evidence:

• Like a tourist using high-school French to ask directions in Paris, psychopaths have trouble putting into words emotional ideas because they are vague and poorly understood. In this sense, emotion is like a second language to the psychopath.

• Psychopaths' thoughts and ideas are organized into rather small mental packages and readily moved around. This can be a distinct advantage when it comes to lying. As psychologist Paul Ekman pointed out, skilled liars are able to break down ideas, concepts, and language into basic components and then recombine them in a variety of ways, almost as if they were playing Scrabble.[17] But in doing so, the psychopath endangers his overall script; it may lose its unifying structure or become less coherent and integrated than if he were dealing in large thought units. For this reason, the competent liar often uses a thin "truth line" to help keep track of what he says and to ensure that his story appears consistent to the listener. "The most mischievous liars are those who keep sliding on the verge of truth."[18]

A Fragmented Truth Line

Although psychopaths lie a lot, they are not the skilled liars we often make them out to be. As I discussed earlier, their speech is full of inconsistent or contradictory statements. Psychopaths may play mental Scrabble, but they sometimes do it badly because they fail to integrate the pieces into a coherent whole; their truth line is fragmented and patchy, at best.

Consider the inmate quoted earlier who said he had never been violent but once had to kill someone. We understand this as a contradictory statement because we treat it as a single thought unit. However, the inmate may have been dealing with two independent thought units: "I never committed a violent offense," and, "I once killed someone." Most of us are able to combine ideas so that they are consistent with some underlying theme, but psychopaths seem to have difficulty doing so. This helps to explain the wild inconsistencies and contradictions that frequently characterize their speech. It may also account for their use of neologisms (combination of the basic components of words—syllables—in ways that seem logical to them but inappropriate to others).

The situation is analogous to a movie in which one scene is shot under cloudy conditions and the next scene—which supposedly takes place a few minutes later—is shot in brilliant sunshine. Obviously the scenes were shot on different days, and the director failed to take this into account when putting them together. Some moviegoers—like some victims of psychopaths— might not notice the discrepancy, particularly if they are engrossed in the action.

One other point about the way in which psychopaths use language: Their "mental packages" are not only small but two-dimensional, devoid of emotional meaning. For most people, the choice of words is determined by both their dictionary meaning and their emotional connotations. But psychopaths need not be so selective; their words are unencumbered by emotional baggage and can be used in ways that seem odd to the rest of us.

For example, a psychopath may see nothing wrong in saying to a woman, "I love you," just after beating her up, or in telling someone else, "I needed to beat her up to keep her in line, but she knows I love her." For most people these two events (statement of love, assault) would be logically and affectively incongruous.

Consider this bizarre statement by a man with a high score on the *Psychopathy Checklist* who served three years in prison for fraud and theft—he tricked his widowed mother into obtaining a $25,000 mortgage on her house, stole the money, and left her to pay off the debt from her meager income as a store clerk: "My mother is a great person, but I worry about her. She works too hard. I really care for that woman, and I'm going to make things easier for her." When asked about the money he had stolen from her he replied, "I've still got some of it stashed away, and when I get out it's party time!" His expressions of concern for his mother were inconsistent not only with his documented behavior toward her but with his stated plans for the money. When this was pointed out to him he said, "Well, yeah, I love my mother but she's pretty old and if I don't look out for myself, who will?"

Where Was I?

It now appears that the communications of psychopaths sometimes are subtly odd and part of a general tendency to "go off track."[19] That is, they frequently change topics, go off on irrelevant tangents, and fail to connect phrases and sentences in a straightforward manner. The story line, though somewhat disjointed, may seem acceptable to the casual listener. For example, one of our male psychopaths, asked by a female interviewer to describe an intense emotional event, responded as follows:

Well, that's a tough one. So many to think about. I remember once—uh—I went through this red light and there was no traffic, right? So what's the big deal? This cop started to hassle me for no reason, and he really pissed me off. I didn't really go through the red light. It was probably only yellow . . . so what was his—uh—point? The trouble with cops is they are—uh—most are on a power trip. They act macho, right? I'm not really into macho. I'm more of a lover. What do you think? I mean, if I wasn't in prison . . . say we met at a party—uh—and I asked you out, and, I'll bet you'd say yes, right?

This narrative was accompanied by expansive hand movements and exaggerated facial expressions—a dramatic display that blinded our interviewer to what was happening. However, the videotape of the interview clearly revealed to everyone—including our embarrassed interviewer—that the man not only had gone off track but had trapped her into a flirtatious exchange.

Psychopaths are notorious for not answering the question posed them or for answering in a way that seems unresponsive to the question. For example, one psychopath in our research, asked if his moods went up and down, replied, "Uh—up and down?—well, you know—some people say they are always nervous but sometimes they seem pretty calm. I guess their moods go up and down. I remember once—uh—I was feeling low and—my buddy came over and we watched the game on TV and—uh—we had a bet on and he won—and I felt pretty shitty."

Psychopaths also sometimes make it difficult for their listeners to understand parts of their narrative. "I met these guys in a bar. One guy was a dealer and the other was a pimp. They started to hassle me and I punched him out," said one of our psychopaths. But was it the dealer or the pimp who was "punched out"?

Of course, minor breakdowns in communication are not uncommon in normal people; in many cases they represent little more than carelessness or a momentary lapse in concentration. But in psychopaths the breakdowns are more frequent, more serious, and possibly indicative of an underlying condition in which the organization of mental activity—but not its content—is defective. It is *how* they string words and sentences together, not *what* they actually say, that suggests abnormality. By way of contrast, both the form *and* the content of schizophrenic communications are characteristically odd and bizarre. For example, one of our subjects, who later received a diagnosis of schizophrenia, replied to the question, "Do your moods go up and down?" as follows:

> I'm just such a—believer that—uh—that life is so short and that we're here for such a short time and so—so we're all going to die anyway at one stage so then—uh—you—we—pass on to a totally new strata and all the problems of this

world for us are solved and then we have a new set of problems and a new set of joys—whichever one—uh—it's not something I claim to understand.

This reply is odd in both form and content and is difficult to understand. The psychopath's reply to the same question, described above, although tangential and somewhat strange, can be interpreted as being evasive or glib. We can infer some sort of meaning more readily from his reply than we can from the schizophrenic's reply.

It is well known that psychopaths often convincingly malinger—fake mental illness—when it is to their advantage to do so. For example, an inmate I described earlier was able to con his way into a psychiatric unit—and back out again—by slanting his responses to the questions on a widely used psychological test.

A FEW YEARS ago I was asked to consult on a Hollywood feature film about a psychopathic serial killer. The filmmakers had great concern for accuracy and had researched the subject as thoroughly as they were able. But the scriptwriter phoned me one day in near desperation. "How can I make my character *interesting?*" he asked. "When I try to get into his head, try to work out his motivations, desires, and hangups in a way that will make some sort of sense to the audience, I draw a blank. These guys [the two psychopaths in the story] are too much alike, and there doesn't seem to be much of interest below the surface."

In a sense the screenwriter had nailed it: As portrayed in film and story, psychopaths *do* tend to be two-dimensional characters without the emotional depth and the complex and confusing drives, conflicts, and psychological turmoil that make even ordinary people interesting and different from one another. Invariably, psychopaths are depicted as cardboard characters, and while considerable effort is devoted to graphic, gory, riveting, and gratuitous descriptions of what they *do*—Hannibal Lecter, in *The Silence of the Lambs,* overwhelms people with his pompous erudition and eats them when he can—we seldom learn very much about what makes them tick.

To a certain extent, these media depictions may reflect reality.

Virtually all investigations into the psychopath's inner world paint an arid picture. The philosophy of life that these individuals espouse usually is banal, sophomoric, and devoid of the detail that enriches the lives of normal adults.

A particularly revealing illustration of the psychopath's ability to manipulate experienced psychiatrists and psychologists is provided in Terry Ganey's book about Charles Hatcher, who killed at least sixteen people because it gave him a thrill.[20] Following a charge for murdering a six-year-old boy, he was shuttled back and forth between the courts and a forensic psychiatric hospital. Psychiatrists appointed by the court determined that Hatcher was incompetent to stand trial, but the psychiatrists at the hospital considered him competent to stand trial. And so it went, back and forth. After a seemingly endless series of contradictory psychiatric evaluations, Hatcher tired of the game and turned his talents to outmaneuvering the lawyers and the courts.

However, the evidence presented in this chapter suggests that it may not only be the psychopath's skill at manipulation that sometimes makes it difficult for clinicians to evaluate his or her sanity. An interview in which a psychopath's statements are contradictory, tangential, or poorly connected to one another is bound to influence astute clinical judgment. For example, the trial of John Wayne Gacy, the Chicago businessman and serial killer who performed as Pogo the clown for sick children, was marked by contradictory psychiatric testimony.[21] Prosecution experts argued that he was a psychopath and sane, whereas defense experts said that he was psychotic or insane. One psychologist said that he was a psychopathic or antisocial personality with sexual deviation, and that during interviews Gacy's statements were marked by contradictions, evasiveness, and rationalizations and excuses. A psychiatrist noted that Gacy just liked to talk. Under cross-examination the psychiatrist was asked "if Gacy's effusive stream of talk didn't demonstrate loose associations, a characteristic of schizophrenia. 'When Mr. Gacy says on one hand . . . he killed someone and on the next hand he says he didn't do it, is that loose association?' " The psychiatrist replied, "I think that's lying. I think he doesn't remember what he says from one day to the next because he lies."

[p. 338] The jury rejected Gacy's insanity plea and recommended the death sentence.

Gacy's "loose associations" and his contradictory statements and lies may reflect little more than mental carelessness, lack of interest in keeping things straight for the listener, or part of a strategy intended to confuse the listener. However, in the context of the material presented in this chapter, they also may stem from a condition in which continuity among mental events and the self-monitoring of speech are defective, perhaps even disordered: mental Scrabble without an overall script.

This raises an important issue: If their speech is sometimes peculiar, why are psychopaths so believable, so capable of deceiving and manipulating us? Why do we fail to pick up the inconsistencies in what they say? The short answer is, it is difficult to penetrate their mask of normalcy: The oddities in their speech are often too subtle for the casual observer to detect, and they put on a good show. We are sucked in not by what they say but by how they say it and by the emotional buttons they push while saying it.

DURING A TALK I recently gave at a university in California, a linguist in the audience suggested that in some respects psychopaths resemble skilled story-tellers. Both use exaggerated body language and twists and turns in the plot that engage and hold the interest of listeners and "bring them into the story." For many listeners the performance is at least as important as the story. The linguist suggested that, in this sense, psychopaths are effective story-tellers. Even so, the scripts followed by story-tellers generally are more coherent and logically consistent than are those used by psychopaths. Further, the goals of story-tellers include entertainment and education, whereas those of psychopaths consist of little more than power and self-gratification.

Does This Mean They're Crazy?

Contradictory, inconsistent statements! Emotional poverty! I'm sure that by now you are troubled by a nagging question:

Are these people sane? Are we back to the old mad-versus-bad debate?

Following a lecture I gave on psychopathy and language at a psychiatric conference in Florida, a forensic psychiatrist approached me and said, "Your research implies that psychopaths may be mentally disordered, perhaps not as responsible for their behavior as we once thought. Until now, a diagnosis of psychopathy has been 'the kiss of death' for many murderers. Will it now become the 'kiss of life' for them?"

An interesting question. As I mentioned earlier, psychopaths *do* meet current legal and psychiatric standards for sanity. They understand the rules of society and the conventional meanings of right and wrong. They are capable of controlling their behavior, and they are aware of the potential consequences of their acts. Their problem is that this knowledge frequently fails to deter them from antisocial behavior.

Still, some observers argue, psychopaths are deficient in the mental and emotional mechanisms needed to translate their knowledge of the rules into behavior acceptable to society. If they have failed to develop a conscience, are unable to experience guilt or remorse, and have difficulty in monitoring their behavior and its effects on others, the argument runs, then surely they are at a serious disadvantage compared to the rest of us. They understand the intellectual rules of the game but the emotional rules are lost to them. This modern version of the old concept of "moral insanity" may make some theoretical sense, but it is not relevant to practical decisions about criminal responsibility. In my opinion, psychopaths certainly know enough about what they are doing to be held accountable for their actions.

Chapter 9

Flies in the Web

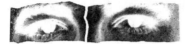

People can be induced to swallow anything, provided it
is sufficiently seasoned with praise.
—Molière, *The Miser* (1668), 1, tr. John Wood

The state policeman stands back as a woman gets out of
her car. He has pulled her over for topping eighty on a narrow
rural road.

It is generally against protocol for a traffic violator to get out
of the vehicle—the standing posture of the officer gives him a
physical advantage and contributes to his aura of authority. And
yet she emerged so confidently, smiled so winningly. She isn't
really beautiful, but the direct eye contact she makes is power-
fully attractive. He asks for her license and resists her attempts
at conversation—for the moment. Finally, though, he gives in
to her bantering style and writes out only a warning. A boy was
killed on this stretch of road only last month, he says. The
officer watches her climb back into her car and drive away,
fighting to keep himself from waving in her rearview mirror.

Most of us accept the terms and rules of human interaction.
But there are always people who use their appearance and
charm—natural or contrived—to convince others to do their will.
And in each case, the "victim's" needs and vulnerabilities help
to determine the outcome of the exchange. Mostly, the outcomes
are relatively harmless, part of the everyday interactions among
people.

But in cases where a psychopath is involved, the impact on the victim can be catastrophic. Psychopaths tend to see any social exchange as a "feeding" opportunity, a contest, or a test of wills, in which there can be only one winner. Their motives are to manipulate and take, ruthlessly and without remorse.

Showtime

As I discussed earlier, although psychopaths may talk a lot they are not necessarily skilled wordsmiths. It is primarily the "show," not eloquent use of language, that attracts our attention and cons us. Good looks, a touch of charisma, a flood of words, contrived distractions, a knack for knowing which buttons to press—all these can go a long way toward obscuring the fact that the psychopathic presentation is nothing more than a "line." A good-looking, fast-talking psychopath and a victim who has "weak spots" is a devastating combination. If the psychopath's "show" is not enough, the adroit use of "stage props"—phony credentials, flashy car, expensive clothes, a sympathy-inducing role, and so forth—will usually complete the job.

Of course, psychopaths are not the only ones capable of theatrical displays. We all know people who are always "on stage," flamboyant, given to the use of verbal and gestural exaggerations and gimmicks. Many of their interactions with others are no doubt shallow and insincere, designed to make a good impression, bolster a poor self-image, or achieve professional or political goals. But unlike psychopaths, their intention is not simply to suck others dry.

Society runs on trust, and we ordinarily pay more attention to what someone says than to the accompanying nonverbal behavior—hand gestures, facial movements, smiles, eye contact. However, when the speaker is attractive and gives a really impressive nonverbal performance, the effect can be reversed—we watch the show and pay little attention to what is said.[1]

THE "PROPS" USED by some imposters seem bizarre, even stupid, to most people, but there is no shortage of eager believers. For six years Ed Lopes, fifty-six years old, posed as a

Baptist minister who had found God on death row. Lopes claimed to have had a fifteen-year career as a mafia hit man for Murder, Inc., during which he had executed twenty-eight people. Nevertheless, he told his flock, and other church groups throughout Washington State, that he had been counseled by Billy Graham, and that petitions from 350 prison employees persuaded the parole board to let him go free. Recently unmasked, Lopes admitted to being a parole jumper from Illinois who had strangled his second wife, beaten to death another woman, and stabbed and choked a girlfriend. His congregation's response? Some members were upset, but others raised his bail, set at a surprisingly low $5,000, and rallied to his support. The court quickly had second thoughts about the low bail and returned him to jail to await proceedings for return to Illinois. [from the *Associated Press*, January 8 and 10, 1992]

Again, psychopaths often make effective use of body language when they speak, and often it is hard not to follow their actions with our eyes. Psychopaths also tend to intrude into our personal space—for example, by means of intensive eye contact, leaning forward, moving closer, and so forth. Overall, their display can be so dramatic or unnerving that it serves to distract, impress, control, or intimidate us, drawing our attention away from what is actually being said. "I didn't follow everything he said, but he said it so beautifully. He has such a gorgeous smile," said a woman who had been bilked by one of the psychopaths we studied.

One of my former colleagues, trapped in a web of passion and deceit spun by a wife he was sure was a psychopath, stated, "She made my life a hell but I feel bereft without her. She was always doing something exciting, outrageous even. She would disappear for weeks at a time, without ever really explaining where she had been. We went through just a load of money—all my savings, the mortgage on the house. But she made me feel really alive. My mind was always messed up when she was around. I couldn't think clearly about anything but her." The marriage ended painfully for him when she moved in with another man. "She didn't even leave a note," he told me.

Buttons

If you have any weak spots in your psychological makeup, a psychopath is sure to find and exploit them, leaving you hurt and bewildered. The examples below illustrate the uncanny ability of psychopaths to detect our vulnerabilities and to push the right buttons.

- In an interview, one of our psychopaths, a con artist, said candidly, "When I'm on the job the first thing I do is I size you up. I look for an angle, an edge, figure out what you need and give it to you. Then it's pay-back time, with interest. I tighten the screws."

- William Bradfield, the psychopathic teacher I described earlier, "never stalked attractive women. . . . [He] could smell insecurity and loneliness the way a pig smells truffles."[2]

- In a chilling auditorium scene in the movie *Cape Fear*, the psychopathic character played by Robert DeNiro mesmerizes and practically seduces a fifteen-year-old girl by playing on her awakening sexuality.

The callous use of the lonely is a trademark of psychopaths. One of our subjects used to seek out depressed, unhappy women at singles' bars. After moving in with one of these women, he convinced her that she needed a car, and sold *his* to her for four thousand dollars. He promptly took off before the formal transfer of ownership could be made—with the car, of course. She was too embarrassed to press charges.

Some psychopaths, particularly those in prison, initially contact their victims through the lonely-hearts columns. Letters often lead to visits and, inevitably, to disillusionment and pain for the victims. Several years ago one of my former students, a lover of Siamese cats, put an ad in a lonely-hearts column, and several replies came from prison inmates, including a psychopath whom she had previously interviewed as part of our research on psychopathy. The prose in his letter was flowery, full

147

of syrupy descriptions of warm sunsets, long walks in the rain, loving relationships, the beauty and mystery of Siamese cats, and so forth, all of which stood in stark contrast to his documented record of violence toward both sexes.

• Psychopaths have no hesitation in making use of people's need to find a purpose in their lives, or in preying on the confused, the frail, and the helpless. One of our subjects carefully studied newspaper obituaries, looking for elderly people who had just lost a spouse and who had no remaining family members. In one case, posing as a "grief counselor," he persuaded a seventy-year-old widow to give him power of attorney over her affairs. His scheme fell apart only because an alert church minister became suspicious, checked up on the impostor, and learned that he was a convicted swindler out on parole. "She was lonely, and I was attempting to bring some joy into her life," said our subject.

• Psychopaths recognize and turn to their own advantage the "hang-ups" and self-doubts that most people have. In his book *The Silence of the Lambs* [pp. 20–22], Thomas Harris describes a revealing scene in which Dr. Hannibal Lecter—"a pure sociopath"—quickly and skillfully manages to detect and use to his advantage FBI agent Starling's weak spot: her fear of being "common."

Agent Starling was a novice at dealing with psychopaths, but even those familiar with the disorder have buttons that can be pressed. Virtually every psychiatrist, social worker, nurse, or psychologist who has worked for any length of time in a mental hospital or prison knows of at least one staff member whose life was turned upside down by a psychopathic patient or inmate. In one case a staff psychologist with a solid professional reputation—and a nonexistent social life—ran off with one of her psychopathic patients. Two weeks later, after cleaning out her bank account and charging the maximum on her credit cards, he dumped her. Her career ruined and her dreams of a loving relationship shattered, she told an interviewer that her life had been empty and that she simply had succumbed to his blandishments and promises.

• Psychopaths have an uncanny ability to spot and use "nurturant" women—that is, those who have a powerful need to help or mother others. Many such women are in the helping professions—nursing, social work, counseling—and tend to look for the goodness in others while overlooking or minimizing their faults: "He's got his problems but I can help him," or, "He had such a rough time as a kid, all he needs is someone to hug him." These women will usually take a lot of abuse in their belief that they can help; they are ripe for being left emotionally, physically, and financially drained.

One of my favorite anecdotes is about a psychopathic offender—a "nurturance-seeking missile"—who had a local reputation for attracting a steady stream of female visitors. His record of violence against members of both sexes was long, and he was not particularly good-looking or very interesting to talk to. But he had a certain cherubic quality that some women, staff included, seemed to find attractive. One woman commented that she "always had an urge to cuddle him." Another said that "he needs mothering."

Deadly Attraction

I have always been puzzled by the strong attraction that many people feel toward criminals. I suppose that in many cases we vicariously live out our fantasies through the actions of those willing to cross over to the wrong side of the law. These "liberated" souls often become folk heroes or role models for people too inhibited to act out their own fantasies of "badness." Of course, most people are generally pretty selective about the folk heroes they choose. Pedophiles, petty thieves, and insane offenders are less likely to fill the bill than are rebels-on-the-run, like those portrayed in movies such as *Bonnie and Clyde* and *Thelma and Louise.*

Perhaps the most bizarre example of deadly attraction is found during and after the trial of a notorious killer: the emergence of a host of courtroom groupies, pen pals, avid supporters, and love-struck fans. For these "desperado junkies," the most powerful attraction of all is to psychopathic serial killers whose savage crimes are sex-related. Ted Bundy, Kenneth Bianchi, John Gacy, and Richard Ramirez, to give but a few examples, all had their enthusiastic cheering sections. In such cases, notoriety is confused with fame, and even the most callous criminal is turned into a celebrity. We now have serial-killer comic books, boardgames, and trading cards, the latter once reserved for sports heroes.

In a book about Richard Ramirez, the Satan-worshipping "Night Stalker," the author described a young co-ed who sat through the pretrial hearings and sent love letters and photographs of herself to Ramirez. "I feel such compassion for him. When I look at him, I see a real handsome guy who just messed up his life because he never had anyone to guide him," she is reported to have said.[3]

Daniel Gingras, a psychopathic killer serving three life sentences in Canada for murder and sexual assault, convinced the prison staff that he should receive a day parole. He escaped custody and killed two people before he was recaptured. A woman from California read about the case, began corresponding with Gingras, and stated that she wished to marry him. "I just saw this picture of him and I had this compassion," she said.

It is difficult for most of us to understand how some people can disregard the monstrous crimes committed by the killers they so admire. What is clear, however, is that these devoted admirers are often victims of their own psychological hang-ups. Some participate because of a romantic need for unrequited love, others because of the notoriety, titillation, or vicarious danger they experience, and still others because they see a cause worth fighting for, such as abolition of the death penalty, a soul to be saved, or the firm belief that the crimes were an inevitable result of physical or emotional abuse in childhood.

It is not only notorious males convicted of violent crimes who attract such avid followers, as the saga of Lawrencia Bembenek illustrates. Nicknamed "Bambi" by the media, she is a former Playboy bunny and ex-cop convicted of the murder of her husband's former wife in Milwaukee. While she was in prison, hundreds marked her birthday with parties in the Grand Hotel ballroom. Following her escape from prison a rally held to celebrate the event drew three hundred people, waving signs that read, RUN, BAMBI, RUN. She fled to Canada, where she was soon recaptured. An extradition request by the United States resulted in an interminable series of hearings, delays, and fawning support from a vocal segment of the public that accepted—and promoted—her claim to be an innocent victim of a frame-up by a male-dominated system. The Canadian authorities considered and rejected her submission that she was a political refugee on the run from American injustice, and she was returned to the United States.

Although she has attained a certain cult status and is the subject of many magazine articles, television programs, and several sympathetic books (one of which she wrote),[4] the Milwaukee authorities insisted that she was in fact an ice-cold killer, a cunning femme fatale. Guilty or innocent, media accounts represented her case as a telling example of "using what you've got" and of society's mindless attraction to the glamorous and the beautiful. Recently, her original conviction was overturned and a new trial was ordered. She pleaded "no contest" to a lesser charge, was sentenced to time already served, and then released. She became a popular talk-show guest.

Bambenek's rise to fame was painfully slow compared to Amy Fisher's leap into the spotlight. Dubbed the "Long Island Lolita," she was convicted of shooting her alleged boyfriend's wife in the head, rapidly became a media event, and was the subject of three television movies, two presented on the same night. A disgruntled "professional" criminal who took part in one of our research projects commented, "She's a nobody. Then she tries to blow away her boyfriend's wife and *botches* the job. Now she's a big star."

In most cases the adulation given to those convicted of notorious crimes is harmless enough; the criminal is seldom helped, and the zealots are not put in real danger, at least as long as the focus of their ardor remains in prison. Rather than being victims of a psychopath's manipulative skills, they are willing participants in a macabre dance.

Distorting Reality

Beyond this vicarious—and generally safe—experience of the dark side of human nature, the sad fact is that the psychopath's need for self-gratification is often easily satisfied because some people are quite willing to play the role of victim. In some cases, the individual simply refuses to believe that he or she really is being taken advantage of. For example, the husband of one of our female psychopaths vehemently denied the credibility of reports from friends that his wife was cheating on him. He remained convinced of her virtue even after she ran off with another man. Psychological denial is an important mechanism for screening out painful knowledge from conscious awareness, but it can also blind us to truths that are obvious to others.

Some people are immune to the truth because they manage to distort reality to make it conform to their idea of what it *should* be. The former girlfriend of one of our psychopaths saw his criminal behavior as an expression of manliness and virility. She looked at him and saw her fantasy of a near-perfect man, "deeply sensitive . . . a mover and a shaker . . . a man not afraid of anything," as she put it. And of course, her projections of who he was fitted in perfectly with his self-image.

Women who rigidly adhere to traditional feminine roles in their relationships with men are in for a very difficult time if any of the men are psychopaths. In contrast, a psychopath married to a woman who has a strong sense of duty to be a "good wife" can have a very comfortable life. The home provides him with a reliable source of succor, a base of security from which to carry out his schemes and to develop an unending series of short-term liaisons with other women. The long-suffering wife usually knows what is happening, but she feels that she must somehow maintain the integrity of the home, particularly if there are children. She may believe that if she tries harder or simply waits it out her husband will reform. At the same time, the role in which she has cast herself reinforces her sense of guilt and blame for the unhappiness of the relationship. When he ignores, abuses, or cheats on her, she may say to herself, "I'm going to try harder, put more energy into the relationship, take care of him better than any other woman ever could. And when I do he'll see how valuable I am to him. He'll treat me like a queen."

IN AN OCTOBER 1991 article for *New Woman* magazine titled "The Con Man's New Victim," Kiki Olson explored an unanticipated side effect of the steadily increasing entry of single women into the professional work force. "The single career woman who has—or can *borrow*—anywhere from $2,000 to $20,000 and is looking for love and money is a natural target for a con man." According to Joseph D. Casey, head of the economic crimes unit of the Philadelphia DA's office, Olson reported, "the male con artist preying on the single working woman with expendable income will stalk his prey in places *she* frequents—singles' bars, health clubs, and social clubs—places where single women congregate, looking for something more than a cocktail, a workout, or a dance. . . . 'The con man will know who she is. He'll be able to spot a certain vulnerability. That's his job.' "

While the women he preys on for money, clothes, room and board, cars, and bank loans are obvious to him in any crowd, the con makes himself indistinguishable from the legitimate suitor. Still, said Casey, "it's safe to say he's good-looking, charming, glib, self-assured, manipulative, and no doubt quite lovable."

In one case, described to me by forensic psychologist J. Reid Meloy,[5] a white-collar psychopath assaulted his wife and seriously injured her. Later, she wrote in a journal she made available to Meloy, "He needs such special care. I haven't been the wife I should have been. But I will, I will, and I'll turn back this anger into something good and strong." This woman's fierce commitment to the man and to being a loyal, "proper" wife had distorted her sense of reality and drained her of all self-confidence. Needless to say, the reality is that she is doomed to a lifetime of disappointment and abuse.

Unfortunately, much the same can be said for any woman— or man—who has low self-esteem, strong feelings of dependency, and a lack of personal identity who becomes intimately involved with a psychopath. Psychopaths have little difficulty in making use of people who feel physically or psychologically inadequate, or who feel compelled to hold on to a relationship no matter how much it hurts.[6]

What Chance Do We Have?

By this time many readers likely have the uneasy feeling that there is little they can do to protect themselves from any psychopath who happens to cross their path. However, even though most of the advantages lie with the psychopath, there are several things we can do to minimize the pain and damage they cause us. (In the final chapter I discuss a variety of survival techniques.)

Chapter 10

The Roots of the Problem

"I know now, so there's no sense in lying any more," said Mrs. Penmark to her daughter Rhoda. "You hit him with the shoe: that's how those half-moon marks got on his forehead and hands."

Rhoda moved off slowly, an expression of patient bafflement in her eyes; then, throwing herself on the sofa, she buried her face in a pillow and wept plaintively, peering up at her mother through her laced fingers. But the performance was not at all convincing, and Christine looked back at her child with a new, dispassionate interest, and thought, "She's an amateur so far; but she's improving day by day. She's perfecting her act. In a few years, her act won't seem corny at all. It'll be most convincing then, I'm sure."

—William March, *The Bad Seed*

The scene described above is from a bestselling novel that capitalized on the unthinkable and "monstrous" idea of children simply "born bad." The novel told the story of a little girl named Rhoda Penmark, whose true nature was revealed in the book when she murdered a classmate:

There had always been something strange about the child, but [her parents] had ignored her oddities, hoping she would become more like other children in time, although this had not happened; then, when she was six and they were living in Baltimore, they entered her in a progressive school which was widely recommended; but a year later, the principal of the school asked that the child be removed. Mrs. Penmark called for an explanation, and the principal, her eyes fixed steadily on the decorative gold and silver sea horse her visitor wore on the lapel of her pale gray coat, said abruptly, as though both tact and patience had long since been exhausted, that Rhoda was a cold, self-sufficient, difficult child who lived by rules of her own, and not by the rules of others. She was a fluent and a most convincing liar, as they'd soon discovered. In some ways, she was far more mature than average; in others, she was hardly developed at all. . . . But these things had only slightly affected the school's decision: the real reason for the child's expulsion was the fact that she had turned out to be an ordinary, but quite accomplished, little thief. . . . with none of the guilts and none of the anxieties of childhood; and of course she had no capacity of affection either, being concerned only with herself. [p. 40–41]

The story told in *The Bad Seed* is really that of Rhoda's mother, Christine Penmark, and it is a story of guilt. Christine Penmark, after forcing herself to see her daughter clearly for the budding psychopath she was, asks herself how on earth the relatively calm, orderly, loving, and promising family life she and her attentive husband had provided resulted in nothing short of a child murderer.

Eerie as it seems, this novel is remarkably true to life. The parents of psychopaths can do little but stand by helplessly and watch their children tread a crooked path of self-absorbed gratification accompanied by a sense of omnipotence and entitlement. They frantically seek help from a succession of counselors and therapists, but nothing seems to work. Bewilderment and pain gradually replace the expected pleasures of parenting, and again and again they ask themselves, "Where did we go wrong?"

Young Psychopaths

To many people the very idea of psychopathy in childhood is inconceivable. Yet, we have learned that elements of this personality disorder first become evident at a very early age. A mother who read of my work in a newspaper article wrote this note to me, clearly in desperation: "My son was always willful and difficult to get close to. At five years old he had figured out the difference between right and wrong: if he gets away with it, it's right; if he gets caught, it's wrong. From that point on, this has been his mode of operation. Punishment, family blow-ups, threats, pleas, counseling, even a run at what we called 'psychology camp,' haven't made the slightest difference. He is now fifteen and has been arrested seven times."

Another mother wrote that her family was being held hostage by the young boy they had adopted several years earlier. As he learned his way around the world and became more aware of his powers of manipulation and intimidation, this child became the chief actor in a chaotic and heartrending family drama. At the time she wrote the letter, the mother had just given birth, and she and her husband were now in fear for its well-being in the presence of their incomprehensible adopted son.[1]

Many people feel uncomfortable applying the term *psychopath* to children. They cite ethical and practical problems with pinning what amounts to a pejorative label on a youngster. But clinical experience and empirical research clearly indicate that the raw materials of the disorder can and do exist in children. Psychopathy does not suddenly spring, unannounced, into existence in adulthood. The precursors of the profile described in the preceding chapters first reveal themselves early in life.[2]

Clinical and anecdotal evidence indicates that most parents of children later diagnosed as psychopaths were painfully aware that something was seriously wrong even before the child started school. Although all children begin their development unrestrained by social boundaries, certain children remain stubbornly immune to socializing pressures. They are inexplicably "different" from normal children—more difficult, willful, aggressive, and deceitful; harder to "relate to" or get close to; less susceptible to influence and instruction; and always testing the limits of social tolerance. In the early school-age years certain hallmarks emphasize the divergence from normal development:

- repetitive, casual, and seemingly thoughtless lying

- apparent indifference to, or inability to understand, the feelings, expectations, or pain of others

- defiance of parents, teachers, and rules

- continually in trouble and unresponsive to reprimands and threats of punishment

- petty theft from other children and parents

- persistent aggression, bullying, and fighting

- a record of unremitting truancy, staying out late, and absences from home

- a pattern of hurting or killing animals

- early experimentation with sex

- vandalism and fire setting

The parents of such children are always asking themselves, "What next?" One mother, with a graduate degree in sociology, told me that at age five her daughter—whom I'll call Susan— "tried to flush her kitten down the toilet. I caught her just as she was about to try again; she seemed quite unconcerned, maybe a bit angry, about being found out. I later told my husband about the episode, and when he asked [Susan] about it she calmly denied that it had happened. . . . We were never able to get close to her, even when she was an infant, and she was always trying to have her own way, if not by being sweet then by throwing a tantrum. She lied even when she knew we were aware of the truth. . . . We had another child, a son, when [Susan] was seven, and she continually teased him in cruel ways. For example, she would take his bottle away and brush his lips with the nipple, drawing it away while he frantically tried to suck. . . . She's now thirteen, and although sometimes she puts on her sweet and contrite act we're generally tormented by her behavior. She's truant, sexually active, and always trying to steal money from my purse."

Adolescent Behavior Disorders and Psychopathy

The American Psychiatric Association's diagnostic "bible," DSM-IV, has no category that captures the full flavor of the psychopathic personality in children and adolescents. Rather, it describes a class of Disruptive Behavior Disorders characterized by behavior that is socially disruptive and is often more distressing to others than to the people with the disorders. Three overlapping subcategories are listed:

- *attention-deficit hyperactivity disorder*, characterized by developmentally inappropriate degrees of inattention, impulsiveness, and hyperactivity

- *conduct disorder*, a persistent pattern of conduct in which the basic rights of others and major age-appropriate societal norms or rules are violated

- *oppositional defiant disorder*, a pattern of negative, hostile, and defiant behavior without the serious violations of the basic rights of others that are seen in conduct disorder

None of these diagnostic categories quite hits the mark with young psychopaths. Conduct disorder comes closest, but it fails to capture the emotional, cognitive, and interpersonal personality traits—egocentricity, lack of empathy, guilt, and remorse, and so forth—that are so important in the diagnosis of psychopathy. Most adult psychopaths probably met the criteria for a diagnosis of conduct disorder when they were younger, but the reverse is not true—that is, most children with conduct disorder will *not* become adult psychopaths. But there is a subcategory of conduct disorder—with "poor social relatedness, little anxiety, high levels of aggression, and other 'psychopathic' characteristics"—that is virtually the same as the disorder defined and diagnosed by the *Psychopathy Checklist* in adults.[3]

More direct evidence of psychopathy in children comes from a recent study conducted at two child-guidance clinics, one in Alabama and the other in California.[4] The children, mostly males aged six to thirteen, had been referred for a variety of emotional, learning, and behavioral problems. Basing their work on the *Psychopathy Checklist*, the researchers, headed by Paul Frick of the University of Alabama, assessed each child for the presence of the personality traits and behaviors described in chapters 3 and 4 of this book. The research teams identified a subgroup of children with much the same pattern of emotional/ interpersonal features and socially deviant behaviors that characterizes adult psychopaths. For these researchers, and for countless numbers of bewildered and despairing parents, childhood psychopathy became a stark reality.

A Difficult Challenge: How to Respond

Most of the children who end up as adult psychopaths come to the attention of teachers and counselors at a very early age, and it is essential that these professionals understand the nature of the problem they are faced with. If intervention is to have any chance of succeeding, it will have to occur early in childhood. By adolescence, the chances of changing the behavioral patterns of the budding psychopath are slim.

Unfortunately, many of the professionals who deal with these children do not confront the problem head-on, for a variety of reasons. Some take a purely behavioral approach, preferring to treat specific behaviors—aggression, stealing, and so forth—rather than a personality disorder with its complex combination of traits and symptoms. Others feel uncomfortable with the potential long-term consequences to the child or adolescent who is diagnosed with a disorder widely believed to be untreatable. Still others find it difficult to imagine that the behaviors and symptoms they see in their young clients are not simply exaggerated forms of normal behavior, the result of inadequate parenting or poor social conditioning, and therefore treatable. All kids are egocentric, deceitful, and manipulative to a degree—a simple matter of immaturity, they argue—much to the dismay of the harried parents who daily must deal with a problem that refuses to go away and even worsens.

I agree that it is no light matter to apply psychological labels to children—or to adults. Perhaps the issue with the most pressing consequences for children is the "self-fulfilling prophecy," whereby a child who has been labeled a troublemaker may indeed grow to fit the mold, while others—teachers, parents, friends—reinforce the process by subtly conveying their negative expectations.

Even if the procedures meet accepted scientific standards, no diagnosis is free from error or misapplication by careless or incompetent clinicians. For example, I read of a case in which a young girl was diagnosed as schizophrenic by a psychiatrist. It was later confirmed that she was actually being starved by her parents; once she received proper care her condition improved dramatically. In hundreds of other known cases, and probably countless unknown ones, incorrect psychiatric diagnoses have had a profound impact on patients' lives. And it's not hard to imagine these consequences being compounded if a misdiagnosis means that other, treatable problems are overlooked.

On the other hand, *failing* to recognize that a child has many or most of the personality traits that define psychopathy may doom the parents to unending consultations with school principals, psychiatrists, psychologists, and counselors in a vain attempt to discover what is wrong with their child *and with themselves*. It may also lead to a succession of inappropriate treatments and interventions—all at great financial and emotional cost.

If you are uncomfortable applying a formal diagnostic label to youngsters, then avoid doing so. However, do not lose sight of the problem: a distinct syndrome of personality traits and behaviors that spells long-term trouble, no matter how one refers to it.

Jason

We recently administered a version of the *Psychopathy Checklist* to a sample of young male offenders ranging in age from thirteen to eighteen. The average score on the checklist was *higher* than it was for adult male criminal populations, and more than 25 percent met our criteria for psychopathy. Particularly disturbing was our finding that the offender with one of the highest scores on the checklist was only thirteen years old. Jason had been involved in serious crime—including breaking and entering, thefts, assaults on younger children—by *age 6*. With one interesting exception, he was clinically and behaviorally indistinguishable from the violent adult psychopaths we have studied. The exception was that he was more open and forthright, less guarded and disingenuous, about his beliefs and attitudes than older psychopaths typically are. Listening to this boy talk was frightening.

Asked why he committed crimes, this product of a stable, professional family replied, "I like it. My fucking parents really freak out when I get in trouble, but I don't give a shit as long as I'm having a good time. Yeah, I've always been wild." About other people, including his victims, he had this to say: "You want the truth? They'd screw me if they could, only I get my shots in first." He liked to rob homeless people, especially "faggots," "bag ladies," and street kids, because, "They're used to it. They don't whine to the police. . . . One guy I got in a fight with pulled a knife and I took it and I rammed [it] in his eye. He ran around screaming like a baby. What a jerk!"

By the time he started school he was used to stealing from his parents and local stores and bullying other children into giving him their candy and toys. Often, he was able to talk his way out of trouble. "I'd just look them straight in the eye and feed them shit. It was great. I still do it. My mother bought it for a long time."

There can be no doubt that society is in for a very rough time from Jason. This is not a youngster whose motivations and behavior are readily understandable—he was not emotionally disturbed, neurologically damaged, or the product of a poor social or physical environment. Unfortunately, everyone who works in child guidance clinics, juvenile services, social agencies, youth detention centers, and the criminal justice system knows someone like him. The questions have remained the same for hundreds of years:

- How are we to understand such children?

- How is society to respond and protect itself while protecting as well the civil rights of these children?

As the signs of social breakdown grow more insistent, we no longer have the luxury of ignoring the presence of psychopathy in certain children. Half a century ago Hervey Cleckley and Robert Lindner warned us that our failure to acknowledge the psychopaths among us had already triggered a social crisis. Today our social institutions—our schools, courts, mental health clinics—confront the crisis every day in a thousand ways, and the blindfold against the reality of psychopathy is still in place. Our only hope is bringing to bear what we know about the disorder as early as possible. Otherwise, we will continue applying Band-Aids to a life-threatening disease, and the social crisis will worsen. (I'll have more to say about this in a later chapter.)

Crime and Violence

The last decade has seen the emergence of an inescapable and terrifying reality: a dramatic surge of juvenile crime that threatens to overwhelm our social institutions. Particularly distressing is the staggering increase in drug use and crimes of violence— homicide, rape, robbery, aggravated assault—and the ever younger age at which these offenses are committed. We are constantly sickened and saddened—but no longer surprised— by reports of children under the age of ten who are capable of the sort of mindless violence that once was reserved for hardened adult criminals.

Psychologist Rolf Loeber[5] draws our attention to the well-known fact that clinical practitioners have never had much luck in rehabilitating youngsters once their antisocial behavior has become entrenched, and that most treatment programs result in little more than short-term gains. Loeber then points to an issue that is often obscured by the sheer weight of the current data on delinquent behavior in our society: "The level of impairment that arose in the 1960s and 1970s in juveniles' functioning should cause concern about the ability of a proportion of that generation to bring up the next generation. Impaired child rearing practices is one of the factors that influence how antisocial a next generation will be." [p. 3] In other words, hold on to your hats—we ain't seen nothing yet.

Loeber notes that there are several well-established pathways to criminality and that it would be illogical and foolish not to do everything in our power to disrupt these pathways as early as possible. The same reasoning applies, with even greater force, to psychopathy.

Ken Magid and Carole McKelvey use the concept of psychopathy to account, at least in part, for the burgeoning crime statistics among the young.[6] To illustrate the point, they present a disturbing list of recent headlines from newspapers across the country:

- Teenage boy in Colorado waits patiently while two young friends hack and hammer his mother to death.

- Florida police try to determine if 5-year-old knew consequences when he threw 3-year-old off fifth-floor stairwell.

- Kansas City police are baffled by jealous 12-year-old who kills younger sister, mother over birthday party plans.

- Eleven-year-old from affluent St. Louis neighborhood orders 10-year-old out of her yard; when he doesn't leave she shoots him with parents' gun. Playmate dies after surgery.

- Girl, 4, kills twin baby brothers by throwing them to the floor after one of the 3-week-old infants accidentally scratches her during play.

I could add dozens of other cases to this list. For example, at this writing a small town in a western state is frantically searching for ways to deal with a nine-year-old who allegedly rapes and molests other children at knife point. He is too young to be charged and cannot be taken into care because "such action may only be taken when the child is in danger, not his victims," according to a child protection official.[7]

These horrific events were not ordinary accidents or simple exaggerations of normal childhood behaviors that will correct themselves with time. Events of this sort begin to make sense when we accept the fact that the personality traits of psychopathy are present early in life. Disturbing as this may be, it paves the way for study of the disorder across the life span, a crucial task if we are to develop effective intervention procedures and to find out what leads one youngster with the disorder to become a con artist or swindler, another to become a violent criminal, another to become a shady or unethical businessperson, politician, or professional, and yet another—perhaps with a less potent mix of the characteristics described in chapters 3 and 4—to become a reasonably productive member of society.

Origins

When we think about psychopathy in children we come very quickly to a single fundamental question: Why? As noted earlier, many adolescents go off track because of a poor social environment—abusive parents, poverty, lack of job opportunities, bad companions—but the psychopath seems off track from the start. Again: Why?

Unfortunately, the forces that produce a psychopath are still obscure to researchers. However, several rudimentary theories about the causes of psychopathy are worth considering. At one end of the spectrum are theories that view psychopathy as largely the product of genetic or biological factors (nature), whereas theories at the other end of the spectrum posit that psychopathy results entirely from a faulty early social environment (nurture). As with most controversies, the "truth" no doubt lies somewhere in between. That is, psychopathic attitudes and behaviors very likely are the result of a *combination* of biological factors and environmental forces.

Nature

Evidence of the genetic and biological bases of temperament, the ability of some forms of brain damage to produce psychopathiclike symptoms, and the early appearance of psychopathic behaviors in children provide frameworks for several biological theories on the origins of psychopathy.

• The relatively new discipline of sociobiology argues that psychopathy is not so much a psychiatric disorder as an expression of a particular genetically based reproductive strategy.[8] Simply, sociobiologists assert that one of our main roles in life is to reproduce, thereby passing on our genes to the next generation. We can do so in a number of ways. One reproductive "strategy" is to have only a few children and to nurture them carefully, thus ensuring that they have a good chance of survival. A different strategy is to have so many children that some are bound to survive, even if they are neglected or abandoned. Psychopaths supposedly adhere to an extreme version of the latter strategy: They reproduce as often as possible and waste little energy in worrying about the welfare of their offspring. In this way, they propagate their genes with little or no personal investment.

For male psychopaths, the most effective way to have lots of children is to mate with—and quickly abandon—a large number of women. Unless a psychopath is so attractive or charming that women actively pursue him, he can best accomplish his goal by deception, manipulation, cheating, and misrepresenting his status. One of our psychopathic subjects, a thirty-year-old fraud artist, has had dozens of common-law marriages, the first when he was age sixteen. He had a peripheral association with several rock stars and often passed himself off as their agent and personal confidant. He had little difficulty in convincing aspiring entertainers that he could give their careers a big boost. In eight cases that I know about, he moved in with such women, and as soon as they became pregnant he left them. Asked about his children, he said, "What's there to tell? They're kids, that's all."

TERRY IS TWENTY-ONE, the second of three boys born into a wealthy and highly respected family. His older brother is a doctor and his younger brother is a scholarship student in his second year of college. Terry is a first-time offender, serving two years for a series of robberies committed a year ago. He is also a psychopath.

By all accounts, his family life was stable, his parents were warm and loving, and his opportunities for success were enormous. His brothers were honest and hardworking, whereas he simply "floated through life, taking whatever was offered." His parents' hopes and expectations were less important to him than having a good time. Still, they supported him emotionally and financially through an adolescence marked by wildness, testing the limits, and repeated brushes with the law—speeding, reckless driving, drunkenness—but no formal convictions. By age twenty he had fathered two children and was heavily involved in gambling and drugs. When he could no longer obtain money from his family he turned to robbing banks, and was soon caught and sent to prison. "I wouldn't be here if my parents had come across when I needed them," he said. "What kind of parents would let their son rot in a place like this?" Asked about his children, he replied, "I've never seen them. I think they were given up for adoption. How the hell should I know!"

Sociobiologists don't argue that the sexual behavior of people is *consciously* directed to passing on their gene pool, only that nature has provided us with various strategies for doing so, one of which happens to be the "cheating" strategy used by psychopaths. When asked if he was promiscuous because he wanted to have lots of children and thus attain a sort of "genetic immortality," one of our psychopathic subjects laughed and said, "I just like to fuck."

The behavior of female psychopaths also reflects a cheating strategy, one in which sexual relations are had with a large number of men and the welfare of the offspring is ignored. "I can always have another," a female psychopath coldly replied when I questioned her about an incident in which her two-year-old daughter was beaten to death by one of her many lovers. (Two older children had previously been taken into protective custody.) When asked why she would want to have another child, given her obvious lack of concern for the fate of her first three, she said, "I love children." Like most of the female psychopaths we study, her expressed affection for children was starkly contradicted by her behavior. Female psychopaths routinely physically or emotionally neglect their children or simply abandon them as they move from one sexual encounter to the next. A chilling illustration is provided by Diane Downs, who abused, neglected, and eventually shot her children, all the while having a prolonged series of affairs. She also became a "professional" surrogate mother, eager to become pregnant for a fee.[9]

Of course, people who make a practice of lying and cheating usually get caught. Their effectiveness then is greatly reduced, so they quickly move on to other partners, groups, neighborhoods, or cities. Their mobile, nomadic lifestyle, and the ease with which they adapt to new social environments, can be seen as part of a constant need for fresh breeding grounds.

One other point. Cheating skills may have adaptive value in some segments of a competitive society such as ours. In other words, far from landing at the bottom of the heap, psychopaths might be helped up some success ladders by their distinctive personality traits.

The sociobiological theory has strong intuitive appeal for some people, but is difficult to test scientifically; most of the supportive evidence is circumstantial and anecdotal.

• A biological theory that has been around for a long time is that, for reasons unknown, some of the psychopath's brain structures mature at an abnormally slow rate.[10] The basis for this theory is twofold: similarities between the EEGs (recorded brain waves) of adult psychopaths and those of normal adolescents; and similarities between some of the psychopath's characteristics—including egocentricity, impulsivity, selfishness, and unwillingness to delay gratification—and those of children. To some investigators, this suggests that psychopathy reflects little more than a developmental delay. Harvard psychologist Robert Kegan, for example, has argued that behind Cleckley's "mask of sanity" lies not insanity but a young child of nine or ten.[11]

These are interesting speculations, but the brain-wave characteristics in question are also associated with drowsiness or boredom in normal adults, and could as well result from the psychopath's sleepy disinterest in the procedures used to measure them as from a delay in brain development. Furthermore, I doubt that the egocentricity or impulsivity of children and psychopaths are really the same. I am certain that few people have difficulty in distinguishing between the personality, motivations, and behavior of a normal ten-year-old and those of an adult psychopath, even after allowing for the difference in age. More important, few parents of a ten-year-old psychopath would confuse him or her with an ordinary ten-year-old.

• An interesting biological model argues that psychopathy results from early brain damage or dysfunction, especially in the front of the brain, which plays a major role in high-level mental activities. This model is based on some apparent behavioral similarities between psychopaths and patients with damage to the frontal lobes of their brains. These similarities include poor long-term planning, low frustration tolerance, shallow affect, irritability and aggressiveness, socially inappropriate behavior, and impulsivity.

However, recent research has failed to find any evidence of frontal-lobe damage in psychopaths.[12] Moreover, the similarities between psychopaths and frontal-lobe patients may be only superficial, or at least no more important than the differences. Still, several investigators have argued persuasively that some sort of frontal-lobe dysfunction—not necessarily involving actual damage—may underlie the psychopath's impulsivity and frequent failure to inhibit inappropriate behavior.[13] It is well established that the frontal lobes play a crucial role in the regulation of behavior, and it seems reasonable to hypothesize that, for some reason—"faulty wiring," early damage—they are relatively ineffective in regulating the behavior of the psychopath.

Nurture

My favorite comic strip is "Calvin & Hobbes." In one sequence an irritated Calvin yells, "Why do I have to go to bed now? I never get to do what I want! If I grow up to be some sort of psychopath because of this you'll be sorry!" "Nobody ever became a psychopath because he had to go to bed at a reasonable hour," his father replies. "Yeah," retorts Calvin. "but you won't let me chew tobacco either! You never know what might push me over the brink!"

Calvin reflects what is perhaps the most popular generalization about psychopathy—that it is the result of early psychological trauma or adverse experiences: poverty, emotional or physical deprivation or abuse, parental rejection, inconsistent disciplinary techniques, and so on. Unfortunately, the picture that emerges from clinical experience and research is far from clear on this matter. On balance, however, I can find no convincing evidence that psychopathy is the direct result of early social or environmental factors. (I realize that my opinion will be unacceptable to people who believe that virtually all adult antisocial behavior—from petty theft to mass murder—stems from early maltreatment or deprivation.)

The neglect and abuse of children *can* cause horrendous psychological damage.[14] Children damaged in this way often have lower IQs and an increased risk of depression, suicide, acting out, and drug problems. They are more likely than others to be violent and to be arrested as juveniles. Among preschool children the abused and neglected are more likely than other children to get angry, refuse to follow directions, and to show a lack of enthusiasm. By the time they enter school, they tend to be hyperactive, easily distracted, lacking in self-control, and not well liked by their peers. But these factors do not make them into psychopaths.

There is little doubt that correction of these early problems ultimately would lead to a dramatic reduction in crime and other forms of social dysfunction. But it is unlikely there would be a comparable reduction in the number of psychopaths and in the severity of their antisocial behavior.

Adorable, Terrifying Tess

In a made-for-television film psychologist Ken Magid is shown working with six-and-a-half-year-old Tess—an angel to look at, with wide, sweet blue eyes and a gap where her front baby teeth have fallen out. The bulk of the film consists of videotapes of therapy sessions with Tess. Hearing her speak of the pain she inflicts on her younger brother Benjamin in the night—to the point where her parents feel they must lock her in her room so that the embattled baby can sleep unharmed—is not only chilling, it conflicts sorely with our understanding of childhood behavior (the children's names have been changed).

"Tess's abuse of Benjamin made life miserable," her adoptive father told the interviewer. "We thought at first Benjamin might have an abdominal problem, but it turned out that Tess was punching him in the stomach at night. We had to tie her door shut."

Tess stole knives—"big, sharp ones," she admitted. "What did you want to do with them, Tess?" Magid asked his small patient. Calmly the little girl answered, "Kill Mommy and Benjamin . . ."

At one point, the film's narrator recounted how, in one of many episodes of violent rage, Tess banged Benjamin's head repeatedly against a cement floor. Her mother had to pry Tess's hands from the baby's head.

"I didn't stop," Tess reported. "I just kept on hurting him."

"Thinking . . .?" the therapist urged.

"Thinking of killing him."

At another point in the video, Magid asked Tess to tell him how she treats small animals.

"Stick 'em with pins. A lot," the girl says. "Kill 'em."

Tess and her brother Benjamin had been adopted by a loving couple who were appalled and frightened by Tess's behavior. In attempting to understand, they researched Tess's case and learned that as babies in their biological family both children, but particularly Tess, had suffered unimaginable sexual abuse and psychological and physical neglect. Magid presented Tess as a vivid—indeed, an unforgettable—example of what can happen to children who fail to "attach" or "bond" to their parents or primary care givers during early life. His book, High Risk, first published in 1987, outlined the position that the failure of the psychological parent-child bond to form at the proper developmental stage, from birth to age two, is a major factor in the development of psychological and behavioral problems, including psychopathy.[15]

Attachment theories continue to be popular in large part because they appear to "explain" everything from anxiety and depression to multiple personality disorder, schizophrenia, eating disorders, alcoholism, and crime. But most of the empirical support for these theories comes from retrospective reports of early experiences, certainly not the most reliable source of scientific data.[16] Moreover, there is little evidence that early attachment difficulties have anything to do with the development of psychopathy.

Most of the external factors associated with the "failure to bond"—rejection, deprivation, neglect, abuse, and so forth—can indeed produce terrible effects, and *some* of these effects may resemble a few of the traits and behaviors that define the disorder of psychopathy.

Certainly little Tess in the television film seems a poignant example. But there is no evidence to suggest that failure to bond can result in anywhere near the full gamut of symptoms comprised by psychopathy—including the characteristic manipulative charm and the distinct *lack* of serious and debilitating psychological symptoms found in those who have been emotionally damaged by their social and physical environments.

While some assert that psychopathy is the *result* of attachment difficulties in infancy, I turn the argument around: In some children the very failure to bond is a *symptom* of psychopathy. It is likely that these children lack the capacity to bond readily, and that their lack of attachment is largely the result, not the cause, of psychopathy.

This possibility is conveniently overlooked by those who assert that a poor environment or improper parenting is everything. The parents of a young psychopath who has turned their lives upside down, in spite of their frantic attempts to understand and nurture him or her, will find it doubly difficult to bear when society unfairly blames *them* for the problem. Their psychological guilt trip to find out where *they* went wrong is not likely to be very fruitful.

An Interactive Model: Nature and Nurture

The position I favor is that psychopathy emerges from a complex—and poorly understood—interplay between biological factors and social forces. It is based on evidence that genetic factors contribute to the biological bases of brain function and to basic personality structure, which in turn influence the way the individual responds to, and interacts with, life experiences and the social environment.[17] In effect, the elements needed for the development of psychopathy—including a profound inability to experience empathy and the complete range of emotions, including fear—are provided in part by nature and possibly by some unknown biological influences on the developing fetus and neonate. As a result, the capacity for developing internal controls and conscience and for making emotional "connections" with others is greatly reduced.

This doesn't mean that psychopaths are destined to develop along a fixed track, born to play a socially deviant role in life. But it does mean that their biological endowment—the raw material that environmental, social, and learning experiences fashion into a unique individual—provides a poor basis for socialization and conscience formation. To use a simple analogy, the potter is instrumental in molding pottery from clay (nurture), but the characteristics of the pottery also depend on the sort of clay available (nature).[18]

Although psychopathy is not primarily the result of poor parenting or adverse childhood experiences, I think they play an important role in shaping what nature has provided. Social factors and parenting practices influence the way the disorder develops and is expressed in behavior.

Thus, an individual with a mix of psychopathic personality traits who grows up in a stable family and has access to positive social and educational resources might become a con artist or white-collar criminal, or perhaps a somewhat shady entrepreneur, politician, or professional. Another individual, with much the same personality traits but from a deprived and disturbed background, might become a drifter, mercenary, or violent criminal.

In each case, social factors and parenting practices help to shape the behavioral *expression* of the disorder, but have less effect on the individual's inability to feel empathy or to develop a conscience. No amount of social conditioning will *by itself* generate a capacity for caring about others or a powerful sense of right and wrong. To extend my earlier analogy, psychopathic "clay" is much less malleable than is the clay society's potters usually have to work with.

One implication of this view for the criminal justice system is that the quality of family life has much less influence on the antisocial behaviors of psychopaths than it does on the behavior of most people. In several recent studies we evaluated the effects of early family background on later criminality in psychopathic and other criminals.[19]

• We found no evidence that the family backgrounds of psychopaths differed from those of other criminals. Not surprisingly, most criminals came from families marked by some sort of problem.

• Among the criminals who were *not* psychopaths, the quality of family background was strongly related to the age of onset and seriousness of early criminal activities. Thus, those from a troubled or disadvantaged family background first appeared in adult court at about age fifteen, whereas those from a relatively stable background first appeared in adult court at a much later age, about twenty-four.

• In sharp contrast, the quality of family life had absolutely no effect on the emergence of criminality in psychopaths.

Whether the family life was stable or unstable, psychopaths first appeared in adult court at an average age of fourteen.

• The findings for the criminals who were not psychopaths are consistent with the general literature on criminality: That is, adverse family influences promote the early development of criminal activity. However, even a good family life that promotes healthy behavior in their siblings does little to deter psychopaths from their lives of callous self-gratification.

• There is one important exception to these general conclusions: Our research indicated that psychopaths from unstable backgrounds committed many more *violent* offenses than did those from stable backgrounds, whereas background had little effect on the violence of other criminals. This is consistent with my earlier suggestion that social experiences influence the behavioral expression of psychopathy. A deprived and disturbed background, where violent behavior is common, finds a willing pupil in the psychopath, for whom violence is not emotionally different from other forms of behavior. Other people also learn violent behaviors, of course, but because of their greater ability to empathize with others and to inhibit impulses, they do not act out as readily as do psychopaths.

Another Look at the Camouflage Society

In view of our increasingly widespread social distress, the issue of psychopathy's origins gains an ominous significance. A recent case in the city in which I live brought home not only the seriousness of rising juvenile crime rates but the meaning behind the statistics. A thirteen-year-old killer was given the maximum sentence under the Canadian Young Offenders Act—three years—for the bludgeoning murder of a twelve-year-old youth. The motive for the murder? The youth had failed to provide $250 worth of marijuana paid for by the murderer—a very grown-up crime indeed.[20]

The unnamed murderer was described as manipulative, street-wise, and "messed up from the start." The details *surrounding* the murder are of lasting significance. For example, friends from the murderer's neighborhood described him as "just 'a regular guy' who skipped school, smoked marijuana and played video games. . . . When asked if the youth had any special interests, his friends said shoplifting. . . . [The] defense lawyer . . . told the bail hearing the convicted killer began breaking into apartments at age eight. The youth was starting fires at age nine and he ran away ten times during the last three years . . . The boy has convictions for breaking and entering, theft and possession of narcotics. He was suspended from school several times for disruptive behavior and truancy. In Grade 7 he was expelled for stealing from the milk program. He smoked marijuana daily by age 11 and later became a regular user of hashish and occasionally cocaine. . . . In his sentencing, [the judge] cited doctors' profiles that say the youth shows classic 'anti-social' behavior. They do not experience guilt in the same fashion as others and have difficulty empathizing . . . by and large they do not change over time."

Sound familiar? Perhaps, although I cannot make a long-distance diagnosis based on a few loosely reported details. The point of this portrait is not diagnosis of the young assailant but rather this comment on the circumstances surrounding his murderous act: "Stories circulating in the [area where he lived] suggested as many as 20 youths knew the accused was responsible for the murder but said nothing."

GANGS HAVE ALWAYS provided great opportunities for young psychopaths. Their impulsive, selfish, callous, egocentric, and aggressive tendencies easily blend in with—and may even set the tone for—many of the gang's activities. Indeed, there cannot be many other activities that produce so many rewards for violent psychopaths, and with such impunity. Local youth gangs are heavily involved in drug dealing, theft, intimidation, and extortion. They recruit many of their new members from the schools, and their presence in and around the schools is a constant reminder to students and teachers of the influence and raw power gangs have.

Although society is showing increased alarm at the presence of gangs in our communities, penalties for unlawful gang-related acts often remain trivial. In a recent case, two fifteen-year-olds and a sixteen-year-old were charged with gang-related activities, including assault, auto theft, possession of a dangerous weapon, assault with a dangerous weapon, and assault causing bodily harm. Most of the charges were dropped because the parents of the teenage witnesses, fearing reprisals, refused to allow their youngsters to testify in court. A police spokesman said that it was "very disturbing that through threats and intimidation a criminal can have the charge against him dropped," and he noted that there is always witness tampering in any gang-related charge. These gangs have a collective sense of power and invincibility that is not unlike that of some of their psychopathic members.

If, as I believe, our society is moving in the direction of permitting, reinforcing, and in some instances actually valuing some of the traits listed in the *Psychopathy Checklist*—traits such as impulsivity, irresponsibility, lack of remorse, and so on— our schools may be evolving into microcosms of a "camouflage society," where true psychopaths can hide out, pursuing their destructive, self-gratifying ways and endangering the general student population. Troubling indeed are the implications of the silence of those twenty Canadian youths who knew of a murder, knew the identity of the murderer, but, whatever their reasons, told no one. They suggest that our society may be not only fascinated but increasingly tolerant of the psychopathic personality. Even more frightening is the possibility that "cool" but vicious psychopaths will become twisted role models for children raised in dysfunctional families or disintegrating communities where little value is placed on honesty, fair play, and concern for the welfare of others.

"What Have I Done?"

It is hard to imagine any parent of a psychopath who has not asked the question, almost certainly with a sense of desperation,

"What have I done wrong as a parent to bring this about in my child?"

The answer is, possibly nothing. To summarize our sparse data, we do not know why people become psychopaths, but current evidence leads us away from the commonly held idea that the behavior of parents bears sole or even primary responsibility for the disorder. This does not mean that parents and the environment are completely off the hook. Parenting behavior may not be responsible for the essential ingredients of the disorder, but it may have a great deal to do with how the syndrome develops and is expressed. There is little doubt that poor parenting and unfavorable social and physical environments can greatly exacerbate potential problems and that they play a powerful role in molding the behavioral patterns of children. The complex interplay of these forces helps to determine why only a few psychopaths become serial killers while the vast majority go through life as "ordinary" criminals, shady businessmen, or legal predators.

Although the origins of psychopathy remain murky, the improved accuracy in diagnosis and the growing body of research allow us to begin formulating better ways to deal with the psychopaths in our communities. That is the subject of this book's final chapters.

IN 1981, IN Milpitas, California, thirteen teenagers kept silent for three days after a boy murdered a fourteen-year-old girl in their class. During that period the group made trips into the hills to view the body. *River's Edge,* a 1987 movie based on the facts of the case, depicts those children as members of a "blank generation." To anyone acquainted with the current communication styles of some teenagers, the portrayal will seem alarmingly familiar. This skillfully made film offers unusual insight into the ways in which a lawless subculture of the young can be camouflaged.

The world these children inhabit is a white working-class neighborhood of a type rarely depicted realistically in films. There, children drenched in television violence form a secret underworld while their parents struggle to make ends meet and their family lives spin out of control. Distracted and distressed by the grind of daily life, at best the parents in the movie manage to shout, "Is that you?" to their children as they pass in and out of the house and go their separate ways.

One of the movie's most powerful scenes shows a teacher, still able to care, trying to get through the "cool," ironic style that masks these kids. He asks, then practically begs, the class to say something about how the loss of their dead classmate affected them. Only the "nerd" in the class is willing to admit to caring at all; the rest seem hopelessly confused by the question. Desperately seeking some evidence that he's reaching his students on a meaningful level, the teacher turns to one of them, a girl named Clarissa who was one of those who finally told the authorities of the murder: "Say what Jamie *meant* to you . . ." The response, even from this girl, is a flat, empty stare. Whether the girl had no feelings or refused to divulge them to an authority figure the filmmakers leave to the audience.

The absence of empathy, compassion, or even comprehension of loss drives this teacher into a fit of fury: "Nobody in this classroom gives a damn that she's dead. . . . It gives us a chance to be morally superior but nobody in this classroom really gives a shit that she's dead. Because if we did we wouldn't be here, we'd be out on the street half-crazed from lack of sleep tracking down the guy who killed her."

The chilling response to the teacher's outburst? Silence.

It's just a movie, true. But the portrayal in *River's Edge* of a society where emotional poverty, impulsivity, irresponsibility, self-aggrandizement, and self-gratification are the norms rings frighteningly true. Whereas, as Robert Lindner put it in 1944, frontiers and borders once drew the psychopath with the "sparkle and glitter of personal freedom," today our streets, our schools, and even our homes might afford the psychopath the chance to blend in undetected, undiagnosed, and actively encouraged. I hope that this book will draw attention to this frightening possibility by putting psychopathy in children into bold relief.

Chapter 11

The Ethics
of Labeling

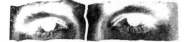

I was kicked out of school in eighth grade for beating up
the teacher. The social worker said, "He's disadvantaged.
Send him to summer camp." When I was seventeen I was
charged with rape. The psychiatrist said, "He's a psychopath. Send him to jail." It ruined my life. They thought I
was rotten so I proved them right.
—A convicted serial rapist who committed his first violent
sexual offense at age eleven

Throughout this book I have argued that precise assessments of psychopathy are essential if we are to increase our
understanding of this socially devastating disorder. But there is
an even more pressing need for accuracy in diagnosis: Before
we can develop effective management and treatment programs
for psychopaths we must correctly identify them.

With our crime rates and prison populations spiraling out of
control, with mental health facilities growing packed beyond capacity, with unprecedented trends in violent crime, substance
abuse, unwanted pregnancy, and suicide surfacing among our
youth, I firmly believe that mental health and social work professionals sorely need to use the concept of psychopathy to guide
their decision making. Properly used, the diagnosis of psychopa-

thy has the potential to clear up some of the confusion about how and why our social order is in such difficulty. However, improper use of the label has powerful destructive potential for the misdiagnosed individual. It is for these reasons that the *Psychopathy Checklist* is such a valuable tool. Not only does it provide clinicians and decision makers with a reliable and valid diagnostic procedure, it provides others—including members of the criminal justice system—with a detailed description of precisely what goes into a diagnosis of psychopathy. Rather than having a clinician simply say, "In my professional opinion this individual is a psychopath," the reasons for the diagnosis are clearly spelled out.

AT A RECENT professional meeting, a prison psychologist told me that the institutions in his state routinely use the *Psychopathy Checklist* to keep the "blame line" for poor parole decisions from reaching them. "It helps us in our recommendations to the parole board," he said. "We tell the board whether or not an offender is a psychopath and explain the implications of the diagnosis. It's then up to the board to decide how to use the information. If he's a psychopath and they let him out and he kills someone, we're off the hook and the parole board has to do the explaining to the public and the victim's family. If he's not a psychopath and all the other evidence indicated he was a good risk and he kills someone, we're still okay. So is the parole board. We all did the best we could, and no parole is without risk."

The psychologist also said that it was only a matter of time until the family of someone killed by a parolee sued the state on the grounds that it had released "a psychopathic killer who had not been properly diagnosed." The *Psychopathy Checklist*, he said, was useful insurance against such a claim.

Only the Parole Board Was Surprised

The public is often perplexed when a criminal with a long record receives what seems an unusually early release from prison. The reasons vary, but in most cases the parole board feels that the offender no longer poses a significant threat to society. In most cases their decisions are sound, but occasionally they make inexplicable and tragic mistakes. For example, consider the case of Carl Wayne Buntion, described on the television show *A Current Affair*, May 7, 1991. He was released from a Texas prison in 1990, fifteen months after receiving a fifteen-year sentence for sexual assault. Six weeks later he shot and killed a police officer during a routine traffic stop.

Why was this man paroled so soon after beginning a long sentence for a violent crime? After all, it was not as if this had been his only crime. His record went back at least to 1961, and he had consistently violated his paroles, which he seemed to get rather easily and quickly. Indeed, in 1984 he was sentenced to two concurrent ten-year terms, but he was out on his seventh parole by 1986. When asked, "How can you say a man with this record is not a threat to society? Clearly this man is a repeat offender," the chairman of the parole board replied, "That's a matter of judgement." He also said that the parole board did not share any of the blame for the police officer's death—"No more than his mother should be blamed for bearing him [Buntion] as a son."

Buntion's girlfriend described him this way: "He is intelligent, he has a wonderful sense of humor, he is very easygoing, very laid back; he is a gentleman." Neither the victim of his sexual assault nor the family of the murdered officer is likely to agree with this rather bizarre depiction of a grossly antisocial man. As television reporter David Lee Miller put it, "Love may be blind, but what's the excuse for the Texas Parole Board for failing to see the truth about Carl Wayne Buntion?"

Is Buntion a psychopath? Probably. Had the institutional authorities insisted that a proper assessment be made as part of his application for parole, and had the parole board been astute enough to integrate the diagnosis and his criminal record, it is unlikely that Buntion would have been released from prison. After all, it would not have taken a genius to predict that a Carl Buntion was not suddenly going to become a model citizen.

However, the sad fact is that parole boards are more likely to be composed of political appointees who have few relevant qualifications than of people who understand criminal behavior and appreciate the potent role of psychopathy in the prediction of recidivism and violence. Moreover, board members often have too little time to do a thorough job. And in many cases they are reluctant to use, or are confused by, the clinical reports provided by psychiatrists and psychologists. Having seen my share of such reports, I understand why many parole boards do not find them very helpful in making difficult decisions about early release from prison. Many clinical reports are vague or full of jargon, and some provide diagnoses that lack empirical evidence of their ability to predict recidivism and violence.

The Power of Labeling

Accurate diagnoses that also have predictive validity can be extremely useful to the criminal justice system. The success of the *Psychopathy Checklist* in predicting recidivism and violence attests to this. However, it is also important to understand the dangers of inaccurate diagnosis and faulty labeling. In the correctional system, for example, a single entry in a file by an intake officer or a prison psychologist can mark an inmate like Cain. Suppose, for example, that a young man in prison for a series of burglaries has become eligible for parole. The overworked and underpaid prison psychologist gives the man a brief interview and makes a cursory examination of his file, noting that a few years earlier a psychiatrist had said that he was an "antisocial personality." In writing his report, the psychologist states that, in his clinical opinion, the inmate is a *psychopath* and therefore a poor parole risk. Parole is denied by a board swayed by what it thinks the label means and concerned about the rising crime rate. The inmate subsequently becomes depressed and commits suicide. At the inquest, the hapless psychologist testifies that he made his diagnosis on the basis of file information and a fifteen-minute interview.

On the other side of the issue, however, *accurate* assessments can be very useful in the classification of offenders, determining work assignments, making decisions about appropriate treatments and interventions, planning for release, and preparing staff to deal with offenders on a daily basis. A diagnosis of

psychopathy also might prevent an offender from being transferred from a prison to a forensic psychiatric hospital (a hospital
for mentally disordered criminals), where he or she would have
a disruptive influence on the other patients. Or, once in such a
hospital, the diagnosis might help determine the security level
at which the offender is placed. In a recent example, a patient
killed a member of the staff of the largest hospital for mentally
disordered offenders in North America.[1] The administration and
staff met and agreed on the institution of a new policy: A patient
with both a high score on the *Psychopathy Checklist* and a history
of violence must undergo a special administrative review before
being considered for assignment to a lower level of security
within the hospital. The review assists staff in the difficult and
nerve-racking task of trying to strike a reasonable balance between the need to reduce violence and the needs and rights of
each patient to receive appropriate treatment.

MOST JURISDICTIONS around the world consider psychopaths
legally and psychiatrically sane. However, in a recent case in
Australia the authorities decided that the only way to keep Garry
David, "an aggressive psychopath," from being released from
prison was to bring in legislation declaring him and others like
him mentally ill. After learning of David's long history of law-
breaking and violence, a Supreme Court judge who heard the
case was quoted as saying, "Someone with such a history
must be suffering from a mental illness and if psychiatrists fail
to realize this they must be 'crazy' themselves." In spite of vocal
opposition from the psychiatric community, David was certified
mentally ill and detained in a high-security psychiatric hospital.
(From Neville Parker. The Garry David case. *Australian and
New Zealand Journal of Psychiatry* 25, 1991, 371–74.)

Long-Distance Diagnosis

In one of life's more satisfying coincidences, I received a call
from CBS asking me to comment on a possible link between
psychopathy and the personality of Iraqi president Saddam Hussein. The Persian Gulf War was at its height, and the general

population was swamped night and day by images and commentary on every aspect of the hostilities and the politics generating them. Predicting Hussein's next move had become a global obsession, and CBS had apparently decided to temper the fervor with some "expert opinion."

I declined the invitation. Like the top-of-the-head diagnosis furthered by "Dr. Death" (described in the following pages), the long-distance diagnosis of public figures, even by experienced diagnosticians, can easily become a parody of professional procedure. The result can be a form of glorified gossip, lent credence not by the facts but merely by the expert's credentials.

In the case of Saddam Hussein, the dangers were especially evident, since, as we were apt to hear repeatedly during the early days of the war, "The first victim of war is the truth." Not only were biographical materials on Hussein limited, but the highly influential variables of culture, religion, and other components of a belief system profoundly different from ours called for careful study and understanding from anyone attempting a psychological diagnosis.

During that same period, Daniel Goleman reported on remarks by Dr. Jerrold Post, professor of psychiatry and politics at George Washington University ("Experts Differ on Dissecting Leaders' Psyches from Afar," *The New York Times,* January 19, 1991, p. C1 ff). In testimony to the U.S. Senate, Dr. Post depicted the Iraqi president as suffering from " 'malignant narcissism,' a severe personality disorder that leaves him grandiose, paranoid and ruthless." Even lay people got in on the act. Appearing on CNN on February 13, 1991, Representative Robert Dornan described Hussein as "sociopsychopathic."

In his *New York Times* article, Goleman went on to show that psychological profiles of public figures have their roots in Freudian theories and have been considered valuable by the U.S. government, but that experts differ in their opinions of their worth. Particularly in the case of Hussein, "critics note that other interpretations are equally plausible, and that [Post's] diagnosis is based on a slim body of evidence."

Nevertheless, Post used his diagnosis both to describe Hussein's psyche and to make predictions about his future actions, stating before January 15, the deadline that former President

Bush gave Hussein for withdrawing from Kuwait, that "Mr. Hussein would probably back down from a confrontation at the last minute."

The facts proved otherwise: Hussein dug in. Post acknowledged that there are limitations to the predictive power of clinical diagnoses: "These are patterns and tendencies. You can say how someone has reacted in past crises, but you can't make hard predictions based on personality alone."

In an interesting twist to the story, an Iraqi who appeared on a February 7, 1991, Canadian Broadcasting Corporation news program said, "Bush wants to kill all Arabs. He is a psychopath."

A MOTHER WHO saw a newspaper article about my work telephoned one day to say, "From the article it looks like my son is a psychopath." She then asked if I would administer the *Psychopathy Checklist* to her son, currently serving three years for theft. I explained that it would not be possible for me to do so, and that, in any case, a firm diagnosis of psychopathy might make it more difficult for him to secure early release. "But that's just the point," she exclaimed. "I don't *want* him to get out! He's been nothing but trouble to us. When he was seven he molested his younger sister. By the time he was nine the police were spending so much time at our home I should have charged them rent. He's in jail now for stealing from his father's firm."

Enter "Dr. Death"

The destructive potential of diagnostic labels in court takes on awesome reality in the figure of Dr. James Grigson, a Texas psychiatrist known in both the popular and psychological literature as "Dr. Death." The most serious category of murder in Texas carries only two possible sentences: life imprisonment or death. Following conviction for such a crime, a separate court proceeding is conducted before the jury to determine the sentence. To decide *for* the death penalty in such a sentencing hearing, the jurors must agree unanimously on three "Special Issues":

1. that the murderer "deliberately" sought the death of his victim
2. that there is "a probability that the defendant will commit criminal acts of violence" in the future
3. that there was no reasonable "provocation" for the defendant's murderous conduct

It is Special Issue No. 2—the question of dangerousness—that usually poses the greatest problem. In an article about Grigson,[2] Ron Rosenbaum wrote:

> This is where the Doctor comes in. He'll take the stand, listen to a recitation of facts about the killing and the killer and then—usually without examining the defendant, without ever setting eyes on him until the day of the trial—tell the jury that, *as a matter of medical science,* he can assure them the defendant will pose a continuing danger to society as defined by Special Issue No. 2. That's all it takes. [p. 143]

The writer went on to recount his harrowing travels with Grigson, who testified in three capital sentencing trials in two days—and whose testimony resulted in a jury decision to execute in all three cases. His description of the doctor on the stand is undoubtedly very worrisome to any conscientious researcher or clinician. Substituting for a detailed examination of the defendant is what's known in legal parlance as "a hypothetical." The prosecutor verbally paints a detailed hypothetical picture of an offender drawn from the defendant's criminal record and other files. Then he asks the doctor, based on that description, "Do you have an opinion within reasonable medical probability as to whether the defendant . . . will commit criminal acts of violence that will constitute a continuing threat to society?"

In the case of Aaron Lee Fuller, convicted of beating an old woman to death and sexually assaulting her corpse in the course of his robbery of her home, Rosenbaum quoted Grigson's answer to the question of whether a hypothetical killer resembling Fuller, the defendant, would kill again:

"What is your opinion, please, sir?"

"That absolutely there is no question, no doubt whatsoever, that the individual you described, that has been involved in repeated escalating behavior of violence, will commit acts of violence in the future, and represents a very serious threat to any society which he finds himself in."

"Do you mean he will be a threat in any society, even the prison society?"

"Absolutely, yes, sir. He will do the same thing there that he will do outside." [p. 166]

And that was it, remarked Rosenbaum. All the "medical," "scientific" testimony the jury needed—in any case all they'd *get*—to justify a judgment that Aaron Lee Fuller was too dangerous to live, beyond hope of redemption, and should be put to death.

Grigson described a defendant as a "severe sociopath" when he gave a positive response to a particular "hypothetical." However, it is apparent that the term is a synonym for *psychopathy* as described in this book.

In an article on the ethics of predicting dangerousness,[3] Charles Ewing noted that Grigson alone testified in this manner in more than seventy capital sentencing hearings, sixty-nine of which resulted in death sentences. He went on to point out that Grigson "is not unique," that juries base their decisions on expert testimony of this kind all across the country.

The United States Supreme Court has upheld as admissible expert testimony by psychiatrists such as Grigson on the condition that the expert state the prediction in language that indicates that it represents *his or her opinion only*. The adversarial nature of the trial system allows such an opinion to be challenged by other experts. But some experts are a great deal more convincing than others. Rosenbaum noted that Grigson, as one of the more flamboyant expert testifiers, has the charismatic power to override any obstacle in the way of convincing a jury that he is right.

Grigson's approach to expert witnessing is unusual, to say the least. Proper diagnostic procedure, as defined by the standards of practice of psychological and psychiatric associations, requires a careful examination and testing of the individual and adherence to widely accepted, reliable diagnostic criteria.

> A FORENSIC PSYCHIATRIST in a southern state recently told me that he was able to argue successfully in court that his client, whom he had diagnosed as a psychopath, was not responsible for a murder because "your research shows that psychopaths suffer from organic brain damage." It soon became clear that he was referring to a recently published neuropsychological study in which we actually concluded that psychopaths *did not* suffer from organic brain damage, as measured by standard tests. His submission to the court on behalf of his client was based on an erroneous reading of our study.
>
> The psychiatrist's mistake was a lifesaver for his client: He avoided the death penalty.

In my view, not only are Grigson's diagnostic procedures and the facile conclusions he draws objectionable on scientific and clinical grounds, but they reflect an odd belief in his own infallibility as a judge of character. Even under the most ideal conditions, with access to high-quality information and using strict diagnostic criteria, psychiatric diagnosis and predictability are not error-free. When a diagnosis has profound implications not only for the treatment but the very life of an individual, we must make certain that it is accurate within acceptable limits. We must also be aware of the fact that even if perfect diagnoses were possible (and they are not), their ability to accurately predict recidivism or violence is limited, simply because the variables that constitute a diagnosis represent only a fraction of the individual, social, and environmental factors that determine antisocial behavior. Nevertheless, there is ample evidence that a careful diagnosis of psychopathy, based on the *Psychopathy Checklist,* greatly reduces the risks associated with decisions in the criminal justice system. Properly used, it can help to differentiate those offenders who pose little risk to society from those who are at high risk for recidivism or violence.

A Tool Is Only
as Good as Its User

The *Psychopathy Checklist* serves a vital function as a descriptive and predictive tool, and clinicians have been quick to adopt it for a variety of purposes. However, having a tool and using it properly are two separate things. The following scenario dramatically illustrates the dangers of failing to use proper procedure in applying this diagnostic tool.

Dr. J, a forensic psychiatrist, well known as an expert witness for the prosecution, testified during a sentencing hearing that, in his opinion, a convicted criminal with several prior convictions for violent offenses presented a continuing danger to society. This opinion was based on the man's criminal record and on Dr. J's determination that he was a psychopath, as defined by the *Psychopathy Checklist,* and therefore unlikely to change his ways. Dr. J's report and testimony were important factors in the prosecution's attempt to have the man declared a dangerous offender and sentenced to an indefinite prison term.

A junior member of a prestigious law firm represented the offender in the sentencing hearing, a decidedly unenviable task given the formidable reputation of Dr. J. As it happens, the lawyer knew a former student of mine, who brought the case to my attention and showed me a copy of the report Dr. J had submitted to the court. I had some reservations about the report, and the lawyer then asked if it would be possible to obtain independent assessments of the offender. Two of my associates, both highly experienced in the use of the *Psychopathy Checklist,* administered the scale to the offender. Each concluded that he was not a psychopath.

I explained to the lawyer, and subsequently to the court, the procedures for administering and scoring the *Psychopathy Checklist.* The lawyer then proceeded to examine Dr. J on *his* use of the *Psychopathy Checklist,* and he soon established that the psychiatrist in fact had not followed the very specific instructions in the manual. Instead, he had used the checklist as a sort of framework to form his professional opinion and to tap the extensive scientific literature that was then available. (This is not an uncommon practice for clinicians; that is, they often use formal diagnostic criteria only as guidelines for forming opinions based on their own clinical experience.) The judge rejected Dr. J's diagnosis of psychopathy and turned down the prosecution's bid to have the offender sentenced to an indefinite term in prison.

The ethical problems addressed in this chapter stem from two sources: the lack of scientifically sound procedures and questionable professional practice. Diagnoses yield sticky labels; faulty predictions based on inaccurate diagnoses can result in confusion and disaster. The antidote to the problem, the preventive against disaster, lies in the careful use of procedures derived from solid scientific research. Anything less is unacceptable.

Chapter 12

Can Anything Be Done?

Dear Ann Landers: I am writing this letter on behalf of my sister who is the stepmother of a 22-year-old high school dropout. I'll call him "Denny." The boy's father was divorced from his first wife when Denny was an infant. He has been married to my sister for seven years.

My sister has spent thousands of dollars on the boy, including $10,000 for a military boarding school, from which he was dismissed for cheating, lying and stealing. She has hired tutors to help him with his schoolwork, taken him to three psychologists who told her he was full of hostility, and had him examined by doctors who ruled out physical problems.

Denny has lived with my sister and her husband, with his grandmother, and with his own mother. He is now living with an aunt. He does not work, does not pay rent and is happy to be supported by anyone who is willing.

My sister and brother-in-law have found him jobs which he cannot seem to keep. They have supported his interest in sports without overindulging him, and now they are out of ideas.

Denny does have some good qualities. He does not drink or take drugs. However, he has been cruel to my sister's dogs and horses. He has been seen kicking and hitting them.

How can this boy be motivated? We fear he will turn to a life of crime unless something is done.

Up Against It in Virginia

Dear Virginia: Why should a 22-year-old work when he can live rent-free and be supported by relatives? Obviously, Denny has been spoiled rotten.

He is an angry, disturbed young man whose life is going to be a litany of trouble unless he is willing to go for therapy and come to terms with himself. It will take a lot of hard work but the rewards will be worth it. The next thing he should do is get his high school diploma.

Show him this column and tell him if he'd like to write, I'd be happy to hear from him.

—Ann Landers, *Press Democrat*, January 8, 1991

I don't know if "Up Against It in Virginia's" sister has a psychopathic "boy" on her hands. But if she does, it would be difficult to find a more characteristic response by a layperson in our society: Quit indulging him and send him for therapy. You might even urge him to write to Ann Landers.

It's a well-meaning approach and one that most people with the financial resources are inclined to take. But where the person in question meets the criteria for psychopathy, it is an approach doomed to failure unless the circumstances and the therapist— and the patient—are very unusual indeed.

More than twenty years ago, in a book directed at psychologists and psychiatrists, I wrote this:

> [With] few exceptions, the traditional forms of psychotherapy, including psychoanalysis, group therapy, client-centered therapy, and psychodrama, have proved ineffective in the treatment of psychopathy. Nor have the biological therapies, including psychosurgery, electroshock therapy, and the use of various drugs, fared much better.[1]

At this writing, in early 1993, the situation with regard to treatment remains essentially the same as it has always been.

Indeed, many writers on the subject have commented that the shortest chapter in any book on psychopathy should be the one on treatment. A one-sentence conclusion such as, "No effective treatment has been found," or, "Nothing works," is the common wrap-up to scholarly reviews of the literature.

However, with our social institutions threatened by soaring crime rates and our legal, mental health, and criminal justice systems overburdened to the point of paralysis, it is essential that we continue the quest for methods to reduce the enormous impact that psychopaths have on society.

CLINICIANS OFTEN DESCRIBE psychopaths as individuals whose powerful psychological defense mechanisms effectively squelch anxiety and fear. Laboratory research supports this view and suggests that there may be a biological basis to their ability to cope with stress. This may sound as if psychopaths are to be envied. However, the downside is that the boundary between fearless and foolhardy is fuzzy: Psychopaths are always getting into trouble, in large part because their behavior is *not* motivated by anxiety or guided by cues that warn of danger. Like individuals who wear dark sunglasses indoors, they look "cool" but they miss much of what goes on around them.

Some particularly gruesome examples of the ability to remain cool in what should be an extremely fearful situation have recently come to light. Jeffrey Dahmer, the Milwaukee man who committed unspeakable crimes, including serial murder, mutilation, and cannibalism, calmly and deliberately convinced police that a naked and bleeding teenager who had escaped from his apartment was actually an adult lover who had been with Dahmer by consent. Dahmer's story was that the two were merely involved in a lover's spat, and the police left, apparently reassured, with the boy still in Dahmer's hands. Dahmer murdered the boy soon after they left. During his trial, in which he pleaded guilty but insane to fifteen murders (the jury found him sane), evidence of other close calls came to light. For example, an *Associated Press* report (February 11, 1992) described an incident in which Dahmer was stopped by police while he was driving the body of his first victim to the dump. When an officer pointed his flashlight at a plastic bag containing the body,

Dahmer calmly said he was upset about his parents' divorce and was taking a late-night drive when he decided to take some trash to the dump. He was allowed to drive away.

Why Nothing Seems to Work

A basic assumption of psychotherapy is that the patient needs and wants help for distressing or painful psychological and emotional problems: anxiety, depression, poor self-esteem, shyness, obsessive thoughts, compulsive behaviors, to name but a few. Successful therapy also requires that the patient actively participate with the therapist in the search for relief of his or her symptoms. In short, the patient must recognize that there is a problem and must want to do something about it.

And here is the crux of the issue: *Psychopaths don't feel they have psychological or emotional problems, and they see no reason to change their behavior to conform to societal standards with which they do not agree.*

To elaborate, psychopaths are generally well satisfied with themselves and with their inner landscape, bleak as it may seem to outside observers. They see nothing wrong with themselves, experience little personal distress, and find their behavior rational, rewarding, and satisfying; they never look back with regret or forward with concern. They perceive themselves as superior beings in a hostile, dog-eat-dog world in which others are competitors for power and resources. Psychopaths feel it is legitimate to manipulate and deceive others in order to obtain their "rights," and their social interactions are *planned* to outmaneuver the malevolence they see in others. Given these attitudes, it is not surprising that the purpose of most psychotherapeutic approaches is lost on psychopaths.

There are other reasons why psychopaths are such poor candidates for therapy. Consider the following:

• Psychopaths are not "fragile" individuals. What they think and do are extensions of a rock-solid personality structure that is extremely resistant to outside influence. By the time they enter a formal treatment program their attitudes and behavioral patterns have become well-entrenched, difficult to budge even under the best of circumstances.

• Many psychopaths are protected from the consequences of their actions by well-meaning family members or friends; their behavior remains relatively unchecked and unpunished. Others are skilled enough to weave their way through life without too much personal inconvenience. And even those who are caught and punished for their transgressions typically blame the system, others, fate—anything but themselves—for their predicament. Many simply enjoy their way of life.

• Unlike other individuals, psychopaths do not seek help on their own. Instead, they are pushed into therapy by a desperate family, or they enter treatment because of a court order or as a prelude to applying for parole.

• Once in therapy they typically do little more than go through the motions. They are incapable of the emotional intimacy and deep searching for which most therapies strive. The interpersonal relations crucial to success have no intrinsic value to the psychopath.

Here's a psychiatrist's dispirited description of psychopaths—whom he refers to as sociopaths—as patients:

> . . . sociopaths have no desire for change, consider insights [to be] excuses, have no concept of the future, resent all authorities, including therapists, view the patient role as pitiful, detest being in a position of inferiority, deem therapy a joke and therapists as objects to be conned, threatened, seduced, or used.[2]

Not exactly the introspective search for personal insight and relief that a therapist hopes to find in a patient. Psychopaths typically want to sit out the psychotherapeutic dance, and many therapists are quite willing to let them do so.

• Most therapy programs do little more than provide psychopaths with new excuses and rationalizations for their behavior and new insights into human vulnerability. They may learn new and better ways of manipulating other people, but they make little effort to change their own views and attitudes or to understand that other people have needs, feelings, and rights. In particular, attempts to teach psychopaths how to "really feel" remorse or empathy are doomed to failure.

These sobering conclusions apply both to individual therapies, in which a therapist and a patient interact one-on-one, and to group therapy, in which people with different problems try to learn from one another and to develop new ways of thinking and feeling about themselves and others.

• As I noted earlier, psychopaths frequently dominate individual and group therapy sessions, imposing their own views and interpretations on the other members. For example, a group leader in a prison therapy program had this to say about an inmate who had scored very high on the *Psychopathy Checklist:* "He refuses to talk about things he doesn't initiate. He doesn't like to be confronted or questioned about his behavior. . . . He refuses to see how he blocks communication and dominates the therapy group by his long-winded monologues that attempt to circumvent discussions about his own behavior." Yet, shortly after this was written, the psychiatrist wrote, "I am certain he has improved. He accepts responsibility for his actions." And a psychologist wrote, "He has made good progress. . . . He appears more concerned about others and to have lost much of his criminal thinking." Two years after these optimistic statements about him, the inmate was interviewed by a female graduate student for one of my research projects. She said that he was the most terrifying offender she had ever met and that he had openly boasted of how he had conned the prison staff into thinking that he was well on the road to rehabilitation. "I can't believe those guys," he said. "Who gave them a license to practice? I wouldn't let them psychoanalyze my dog! He'd shit all over them just like I did."

A FORTY-YEAR-OLD MAN with fifty-five convictions for fraud, forgery, and theft in three countries attempted to avoid deportation from Canada on the grounds that he had been rehabilitated by his friendship with a seventy-six-year-old blind woman. A 1985 psychiatric report had described the man as "invariably pleasant, courteous, intelligent, and engaging," but also as a pathological liar "with an entrenched personality disorder." The immigration department lawyer referred to him as a "pathological liar who could charm the bark off a tree," "a chronic liar ... who could not separate fact and fiction," and a classic impostor. The lawyer pointed out that the man in question was paroled from prison in the United States in the late 1980s, had violated his parole and fled to Canada, and had made his way to Vancouver, "leaving a series of worthless checks across the country." The twist here is that he now claims to have turned his life around because of self-awareness sessions at a Christian meditation center and church led by the woman mentioned above. His claims to have been rehabilitated have been countered by witnesses who testified that he continues to pass worthless checks and that he has not paid his bills. [From an article by Moira Farrow in *The Vancouver Sun*, March 2, 1991.]

Therapy May Make
Them Worse

Some form of group therapy is an important part of most prison and court-mandated treatment programs. Group therapy is sometimes embedded in a "therapeutic community" program, in which the inmates or patients are given considerable responsibility for running their own lives. The ward staff forms an integral part of the community, and is specially trained to focus on the needs and capabilities of the patients and to treat them in a humanitarian and respectful way. Such programs are intensive and very expensive, in terms of both facilities and personnel, and they work reasonably well with most offenders. *But they do not work for psychopaths.*

Evidence for this stark conclusion is provided by several recent studies of forensic patients treated in a therapeutic community program. In each case, the patients were assessed with the *Psychopathy Checklist*.

• In one study, psychopaths were not motivated to do well, dropped out of treatment early, and derived relatively little benefit from the program. Following release from prison, their rate of return was much higher than that of the other patients.[3]

• In another study, psychopaths were almost four times more likely to commit a violent offense following release from a therapeutic community program than were other patients.[4] But not only was the program not effective for psychopaths, *it may actually have made them worse!* Psychopaths who did *not* take part in the program were *less* violent following release from the unit than were the treated psychopaths.

At first glance this finding may seem bizarre. How could psychotherapy make a person worse? But the finding is not at all surprising to those who run these programs. They report that the psychopaths usually dominate the proceedings, frequently playing "head games" with the group leaders and other patients. "Your problem is that you rape women because you unconsciously want to punish them for what your mother did to you," the psychopath pedantically tells another patient. At the same time, he offers few insights into *his own* behavior.

Unfortunately, programs of this sort merely provide the psychopath with better ways of manipulating, deceiving, and using people. As one psychopath put it, "These programs are like a finishing school. They teach you how to put the squeeze on people."

They are also a rich source of facile excuses for the psychopath's behavior: "I was an abused child," or, "I never learned to get in touch with my feelings." After-the-fact insights of this sort explain very little, but they sound good to those primed to hear them. I am constantly amazed at how willing some professionals are to take such statements at face value.

Group therapy and therapeutic community programs are not the only source of new tactics psychopaths use to convince others that they have changed. They frequently make use of prison programs designed to upgrade their education; courses in psychology, sociology, and criminology are very popular. These programs, like those devoted to therapy, may supply psychopaths with little more than superficial insight and knowledge of terms and concepts—buzzwords—having to do with interpersonal and emotional processes, but they allow psychopaths to convince the gullible that they have been rehabilitated or "born again."

Young Psychopaths

Logically, our best chance of reducing the impact of adult psychopathy on society is to attack the problem early. Thus far, however, such efforts have not been very successful. Following an extensive review of treatment programs, sociologist William McCord was led to conclude that "attempts to deflect the person from his or her psychopathic pattern early in life" generally have not been successful.[5] Still, he felt that some hope was offered by programs in which the individual's social and physical environment was completely changed and the entire resources of the institution were mobilized to promote fundamental changes in his or her attitudes and behaviors. But the results of one such program, described in detail by McCord, are sobering. Although the attitudes and behaviors of psychopathic adolescents seemed to improve during and after the program, the effect dissipated as they got older.

The situation may change as we learn more about the roots of psychopathy. Further, psychologists have developed intervention programs that are quite successful in changing the attitudes and behaviors of children and adolescents who have a variety of behavioral problems. Many of these programs deal not only with the child but also with the family and social context in which the problems occur.[6]

If used at a very early age, it is possible that some of these programs will be useful in modifying the behavioral patterns of "budding psychopaths," perhaps by reducing aggression and impulsivity and by teaching them strategies for satisfying their needs in more prosocial ways.

Another Sobering Thought

Virtually all the evidence on the effectiveness of treatment for psychopaths is based on programs for people in prison or psychiatric facilities or in trouble with the law. Many of these programs are intensive, well thought out, and carried out under reasonably good conditions. And still they are ineffective.

Even if some program *were* effective in changing the attitudes and behaviors of psychopaths, there would be no way of using it to deal with the millions of psychopaths not in custody or court mandated to enter treatment. There is little or no chance that any on-the-street psychopaths would even contemplate entering such a program. And society has no means of forcing them to do so.

Occasional case reports or bits of anecdotal evidence claim that some particular procedure has had a beneficial effect on a psychopath. For example, in the past few years several people have told me that they have managed to bring about considerable improvement in the behavior of a psychopath they lived with. They can't understand why I don't get excited about their experiences.

Perhaps they *did* manage to make a therapeutic breakthrough, but there is no way of determining if this is the case. Was the treated individual actually a psychopath? Did he or she improve in middle age, a time when the behaviors of some psychopaths "spontaneously" improve? What was the individual's behavior like before this change? And how do we know that it was the "psychopath" who changed? Many people confuse improvement in the behavior of the psychopath with changes in the way they themselves deal with the person.

For example, a woman with a psychopathic husband may say that he is not quite as bad as he once was. But what really may have happened is that she learned how to deal with the problem by keeping out of his way or by working extra hard to satisfy his needs and demands. She may have buried her personality and sacrificed her needs and aspirations in order to reduce conflict and tension in the relationship.

We cannot take seriously claims of effective treatments for

psychopathy unless they are based on carefully controlled empirical studies.

Should We Simply Give Up?

Depressing though the evidence is, there are several things that we should consider before writing psychopaths off as untreatable or unmanageable.

• First, despite the hundreds of attempts to treat these individuals and the great variety of techniques tried, there have been few programs that meet acceptable scientific and methodological standards. This is an important point, because it means that the evidence we base our conclusions on is not very sound. This applies both to the common reports that a particular program didn't work and to the occasional report that something did work. Most of what we know is based primarily on clinical folklore, single-case studies, poor diagnostic and methodological procedures, and inadequate program evaluation. Indeed, the state of the treatment literature on psychopathy is appalling.

Perhaps the most frustrating thing about reading the treatment literature is that the diagnostic procedures often are hopelessly inadequate or so vaguely described that it is impossible to determine whether a given program had anything at all to do with psychopathy.

Another recurrent problem in trying to evaluate treatment or management programs is the failure to use carefully selected control or comparison groups. We know that the behavior of many psychopaths improves with age, and it is important to know the extent to which a given therapeutic program improves on the "natural" or "spontaneous" changes that occur with age.

• Second, few treatment programs are designed specifically for psychopaths, and those that are have to contend with so many administrative, government, and public policy issues that they soon become something other than what was originally intended. The fact is, a well conceived and methodologically sound program for the treatment of psychopaths has yet to be designed, carried out, and evaluated.

• The third point is that some of our efforts to treat psychopaths may be misplaced. The term *treatment* implies that there is something to treat: illness, subjective distress, maladaptive behaviors, and so forth. But, as far as we can determine, psychopaths are perfectly happy with themselves, and they see no need for treatment, at least in the traditional sense of the term. It is a lot easier to change people's attitudes and behaviors when they are unhappy with them than when they consider them perfectly normal and logical.

But isn't the behavior of psychopaths maladaptive? The answer is that it may be maladaptive for society but it is adaptive for the individuals themselves. When we ask psychopaths to modify their behavior so that it conforms to our expectations and norms, we may be asking them to do something that is against their "nature." They may agree to our request, but only if it is in their own best interests to do so. Programs designed to get psychopaths to change their behavior will have to take this into account or be doomed to failure.

"EVERYBODY SWEARS PSYCHOPATHS can't be treated. That's a lot of hogwash," said Joseph Fredricks, a homosexual pedophile whose long history of violence included the murder of an eleven-year-old boy. "Psychopaths are as human as anyone. They're psychopaths because they are more sensitive than anyone. . . . They can't stand pain of any sort, that's why they let it roll off their backs," he said. [*Canadian Press*, September 22, 1992]

Elements of a New Program

Recognizing the urgent need for new ways to deal with criminal psychopaths, and aware of the prevailing pessimism about traditional treatment programs, the Canadian government recently challenged me to design an experimental treatment/management program for these offenders. I accepted the challenge for two reasons. First, as I indicated above, previous programs typically have been flawed in a number of ways, and none has been firmly grounded in the latest advances in theory, research, and clinical and correctional experience. Second, there obviously is an urgent need for programs that can reduce the likelihood that psychopathic and other offenders will commit violent acts both in prison and following their release into the community.

I put together an international panel of experts in psychopathy, psychiatry, criminology, correctional treatment, and program design and evaluation.[7] At several meetings we decided that the focus of our efforts should be on psychopathic and other offenders prone to violence, and we hammered out the broad outline of a model program that we felt had a reasonable chance of success. The government recently has decided to go ahead with the program, and steps are being taken to set up an experimental unit at a federal institution.

Although it is not possible to provide a detailed description of the program in this book, some broad principles can be outlined. To a large extent, these principles are based on the view that the premise of most correctional programs—that most offenders have somehow gone off track and need only to be *reso*cialized—is faulty when applied to psychopaths. From society's perspective, psychopaths have never been on track; they dance to their own tune.

This means that the program for psychopaths will be less concerned with attempts to develop empathy or conscience than with intensive efforts to convince them that their current attitudes and behavior are not in their own self-interest, and that they alone must bear responsibility for their behavior. At the same time, we will attempt to show them how to use their strengths and abilities to satisfy their needs in ways that society can tolerate.

Of necessity, the program will involve very tight control and supervision, as well as clear and certain consequences for transgressions of program, institutional, and societal rules. It will also take advantage of, and seek ways to speed up, the tendency of some psychopaths to improve "spontaneously" as they reach middle age.

The institutional components of the program will be followed by strict control and intensive supervision following release into the community.

The design of the program will allow for the empirical evaluation of a variety of treatment components, or modules (what works and what doesn't work for particular individuals). Some components may be effective with psychopaths but not with other offenders, and vice versa. The participants in the program will be compared with carefully selected control (untreated) groups of offenders.

A program of this sort will be expensive and always in danger of erosion because of changing institutional needs, political pressures, and community concerns. And it is likely that the results will be modest at best. However, the alternatives—to bear the enormous expense of keeping offenders at high risk for violence in prison, or to run the risk of letting them out—are not very attractive.

If Nothing Works, What Then?

If you are dealing with a true psychopath it is important to recognize that the current prognosis for significant improvement in his or her attitudes and behavior is poor. Even if the experimental program described above bears fruit, it will not be of much use to psychopaths who are not in prison or subject to tight control.

If you are living with or married to a psychopath, you may already suspect that things are not going to get any better, and you may feel trapped by circumstances, unable to escape without putting yourself or others—especially your children—at risk. The problem is particularly difficult—and dangerous—for a woman living with a psychopathic man who has a strong need to possess and control people. Many women may think, "Maybe if *I* change it will be okay. I can try harder, keep out of his way, become more tolerant, give in a bit more." However, as the growing literature on spouse abuse attests, such changes rarely do anything but reinforce and perpetuate the problem.

Of course, the best strategy is to avoid becoming entangled

with a psychopath in the first place. Admittedly, this is a lot easier said than done. But there are some things you can do to protect yourself. If they don't work, the only thing you can do is try to minimize the harm you experience. The next chapter offers some practical advice on both protection and damage control.

Chapter 13

A Survival Guide

The police tell us that a determined burglar can break into even the most secure home. However, they also say that knowledge of how burglars work, common sense, and a good alarm system or an aggressive dog can reduce the risk of being victimized. Similarly, although no one is immune to the devious machinations of the psychopath, there are some things you can do to reduce your vulnerability.

Protect Yourself

• *Know what you are dealing with.* This sounds easy but in fact can be very difficult. Although this book should help, all the reading in the world cannot protect you from the devastating effects of psychopaths. Everyone, including the experts, can be taken in, manipulated, conned, and left bewildered by them. A good psychopath can play a concerto on *anyone's* heartstrings.

Psychopaths are found in every segment of society, and there is a good chance that eventually you will have a painful or humiliating encounter with one. Your best defense is to understand the nature of these human predators.

• *Try not to be influenced by "props."* It is not easy to get beyond the winning smile, the captivating body language, and the fast talk of the typical psychopath, all of which blind us to his or her real intentions. But there are a few things worth trying. For example, don't pay too much attention to any unusually captivating characteristic of people you meet—dazzling looks, a powerful presence, mesmerizing mannerisms, a soothing voice, a rapidfire verbal pitch, and so forth. Any one of these characteristics can have enormous sleight-of-hand value, serving to distract you from the individual's real message.

Many people find it difficult to deal with the intense, emotionless, or "predatory" stare of the psychopath. Normal people maintain close eye contact with others for a variety of reasons, but the fixated stare of the psychopath is more a prelude to self-gratification and the exercise of power than simple interest or empathic caring.[1]

Some people respond to the emotionless stare of the psychopath with considerable discomfort, almost as if they feel like potential prey in the presence of a predator. Others may be completely overwhelmed and intimidated, perhaps even controlled, with little insight into what is happening to them. Whatever the psychological meaning of their gaze, it is clear that intense eye contact is an important factor in the ability of some psychopaths to manipulate and dominate others.

The next time you find yourself dealing with an individual whose nonverbal mannerisms or gimmicks—riveting eye contact, dramatic hand movements, "stage scenery," and so on— tend to overwhelm you, close your eyes or look away and carefully listen to what the person is saying.

Are the eyes "windows to the soul?" Many people believe that they are. Although the eyes are in fact highly fallible indicators of the inner world of others, they are not entirely devoid of information, particularly when the message they convey to others appears inconsistent with the individual's facial expressions and verbal behavior. "When the eyes say one thing, and the tongue another, a practiced man relies on the language of the first," is but one of scores of maxims that could be cited.

An acquaintance told me about her experiences with a "love

thug," a man who had stolen her affections and had then used them to control and batter her emotionally. "I found it difficult to look at his eyes because they confused me. I didn't know what was behind them and they didn't tell me what he was thinking or what his intentions were," she said.

Clinical anecdotes about the "empty" eyes of psychopaths abound, but it is true crime books that offer the most vivid descriptions of how unsettling their gaze can sometimes be. For example, in his book *Last Rampage* James Clarke had this to say about Gary Tison, a convicted murderer who masterfully manipulated the prison system, escaped from prison with the help of his sons, and went on a killing spree:

> But Gary's most striking physical feature—the thing most people noticed and never forgot—was his deep-set, expressionless . . . eyes. It was as if his eyes had no connection with any emotion he expressed. Whatever his mood—whether he was angry, jovial, or anything in between—his eyes remained the same. Empty. It was impossible to tell what Gary was actually thinking or feeling by looking at his eyes. . . . His stare was riveting, unsettling, with a malign intensity. What people remembered most about Gary were those cold, hard eyes. [p. 4]

Joseph Wambaugh's book *Echoes in the Darkness* is about William Bradfield and Jay Smith, two high school teachers convicted (the former in 1983 and the latter in 1986) for killing a fellow teacher and her two children. The book contains numerous references to the eyes of the two men. For example, Wambaugh had this to say about Bradfield:

> He had brooding blue eyes. . . . His gaze was so intense it could transfix, so his blue eyes were variously described as "poetic," "icy," or "hypnotic," depending upon his moods. A colleague reported that "He'd intimi-

date you with those piercing blue eyes. He was so *intense* he could sometimes be spooky." [He] gave his famous stare to Rick Guida (the prosecutor) who'd been told by an FBI agent that the Bradfield stare had once made him fall back two steps. The stare practically demolished Guida. He was literally floored. He sat down and played with [the dog]. . . . When Bradfield tried the stare on a police officer, Jack Holtz, the latter stared back and said, "That bullshit only works on intelligent people."

Equally interesting was Wambaugh's description of Jay Smith, recently freed by the Supreme Court of the Commonwealth of Pennsylvania on procedural grounds. Smith's secretary reportedly said:

You've never seen such a pair of eyes in all your life. There was no *feeling* in them. You might think you've known a few people with cold fish eyes, but not like his.

Wambaugh commented that "They were *not* fish eyes. They were eyes that newspaper editors in later years loved to isolate for effect. They were referred to as 'reptilian,' but that was not correct either." Later he said that *all* the teachers "had trouble describing the eyes of their principal. 'Amphibian' came to mind, but that wasn't precisely correct either."

Smith's secretary finally realized what his eyes resembled, said Wambaugh. "Not fish, not reptiles . . . [but] the eyes of a *goat!*" . . . "That, my friend, is the prince of darkness," said a teacher. [p. 18]

Can the eyes reveal the devil incarnate, as the teacher's comment implies? In cases where a real or fictitious serial killer—a Ted Bundy or a Hannibal Lecter—commits unspeakable crimes it may be difficult to believe otherwise. However, it is likely that the behavior of psychopaths—including the few that murder and mutilate—stems more from a total indifference to the feelings or welfare of others than from sure evil. Their eyes are those of an emotionless predator, not those of satan.

But interesting as they are, anecdotes and examples of this sort should not lull us into the false belief that we can reliably spot a psychopath by his or her eyes. It is all too easy to misread the eyes of others and to draw erroneous conclusions about character, intentions, and truthfulness. To believe otherwise is to court disaster.

• *Don't wear blinkers.* Enter new relationships with your eyes wide open. Like the rest of us, most psychopathic con artists and "love thieves" initially hide their dark side by "putting their best foot forward." But they go further to exploit the axiom that social intercourse depends on trust, and that it is impossible for us to pay close and cynical attention to everything they say and do. Accordingly, they typically attempt to overwhelm their victims with flattery, feigned concern and kindness, and phony stories about financial dealings and social status. Cracks may soon begin to appear in the mask they wear, but once you are trapped in their web of deceit and control, it will be difficult to escape financially and emotionally unscathed.

The police and consumer advocates tell us that extra caution is called for whenever someone or something seems too good to be true. This is good advice and, if followed, will help protect you from the psychopath's potentially deadly snare. At the very least you should take the time to check out any new acquaintance who appears to have a financial or romantic interest in you. I'm not suggesting that you hire a private investigator every time you meet someone at a party or in a bar, only that you make some reasonable inquiries. Ask the individual about his or her friends, family, relatives, employment, place of residence, plans, and so forth. Psychopaths usually give vague, evasive, or inconsistent replies to queries about their personal lives. Be suspicious of such replies, and try to verify them.

This is sometimes surprisingly easy to do. For example, several years ago a woman I know became romantically involved with a man she'd met at her church. He appeared to be well connected and to have impeccable credentials, and he said he was a graduate in business administration from a well-known eastern university. She considered investing heavily in a business venture he was promoting. When I met him I told him that we were graduates of the same university, but he was evasive about his experiences there, always managing to change the subject. My suspicions aroused, I did some checking and learned that he had never been a student at my university. Further investigation revealed that he was a swindler, wanted in several countries. He skipped town, leaving my friend disillusioned by the experience and angry at me for destroying her fantasy world.

• *Keep your guard up in high-risk situations.* Some situations are tailor-made for psychopaths: singles' bars, social clubs, resorts, ship cruises, foreign airports, to name but a few. In each case, the potential victim is lonely, looking for a good time, excitement, or companionship, and there will usually be someone willing to oblige, for a hidden price.

Single travelers are a favorite target of psychopaths, who readily spot them looking lost and forlorn in a foreign airport or tourist spot. For example, I know a professional woman who was weary, lonely, and homesick after several weeks on her own in Europe. She was befriended by a helpful man at the airport in Lisbon. Posing as an undercover agent on the track of a smuggling ring, he managed to win her confidence and to enlist her aid in the operation. In the ensuing weeks the pair traveled all over Europe, running up enormous bills on her credit card. When she finally became suspicious, he dumped her. In retrospect, she said, the whole affair seemed bizarre, but at the time it all made sense. "I was tired, depressed, and he was so understanding and comforting."

• *Know yourself.* Psychopaths are skilled at detecting and ruthlessly exploiting your weak spots, at finding the right buttons to press. Your best defense is to understand what your weak spots are and to be extremely wary of anyone who zeros in on them. Judge such people more critically than you do those who do not seem to be aware of, or catering to, your vulnerabilities.

If you are a sucker for flattery it is certain to be written all over you, an engraved invitation to every unscrupulous operator looking around for fresh victims. Basking in flattery, like sitting too long in the sun, can be pleasant at first but painful in the end.

If you have a bit of larceny in your soul you are particularly vulnerable to schemes that are a bit shady. Lonely people with money are extremely easy targets for the psychopath.

Knowing who you are is not always easy. Self-examination, frank discussions with family and friends, and professional consultation may be of help.

Damage Control

Unfortunately, even the most careful precautions are no guarantee that you will be safe from the predation of a determined psychopath. In some cases, the matter may be beyond your control, as it usually is in an "arm's length" financial relationship with a psychopath. Many frauds and scams are perpetrated against banks, brokerage houses, savings-and-loan institutions, pension funds, and so forth. Individual investors have no say in day-to-day operations, and they can lose their money through no fault of their own. For example, a distraught high-school counselor recently told me about an investment broker who "lost" several million dollars from the teachers' pension fund the broker had been entrusted to manage. The counselor was out several hundred thousand dollars not because he was careless but because the officials responsible for finding a reputable investment broker had been conned by a slick psychopath.

FORENSIC PSYCHOLOGIST J. Reid Meloy tells of his being snared while interviewing an applicant for a job whose entire resumé eventually turned out to be phony. "The interview went quite smoothly, though," Meloy said in a telephone interview. "I was really impressed with this guy, couldn't get over how bright he was. As we talked, he'd drop in a phrase here, a phrase there that really had me standing back and thinking, 'Wow! This guy is actually brilliant. How do I get him to want the job?' It took me a while—longer than I'd like to admit—to figure out that he was quoting from several papers I had written and recently published. He was impressing me, yes, but with what? With my *own* brilliance—ideas of mine I thought a lot of. A normal person might say, 'I read your paper and thought this and such,' but this fellow—who turned out to be a complete impostor—had an intuitive grasp on what among all possible things would get me to do what he wanted. For him the interview was a great opportunity to perpetuate a scam." [personal communication, April 1991]

Perhaps the most heart-wrenching situations are those in which bewildered, frantic parents try to deal with a psychopathic son or daughter. Almost as distressing are those in which someone doggedly searches for a means of coping with a psychopathic spouse. In such cases, as well as those in which a psychopath has managed to enter your romantic life, about all you can do is attempt to exert some sort of damage control. This is not an easy task for most people, but some suggestions may be of help:

• *Obtain professional advice.* I receive many calls from concerned people who think a husband, wife, child, or friend is a psychopath and who want my advice on what to do about it. I cannot offer advice under such conditions. A proper diagnosis of psychopathy, by a knowledgeable clinician, is time-consuming and requires a good deal of reliable information, including an intensive interview with the individual in question and access to collateral and corroborative information from a variety of sources: employers, family members, friends, business associates, the police, and so on.

Make sure the clinician you consult is familiar with the literature on psychopathy and has had experience in dealing with psychopaths, preferably in the context of family therapy and intervention. If you have the resources, *get several opinions.* This can be a very frustrating procedure. I can't count the number of times a telephone caller, usually a wife or parent at wits' end, has described repeated attempts to get someone—anyone—to understand the problem, or even to recognize that there is a problem.

Typical is a telephone call I received from a woman in Maine who had read a newspaper article about my work and was convinced that her husband perfectly matched the profile of psychopathy outlined in the article. From what she told me about him it appeared that she might very well have been right. For more than ten years she had been trying to get professional help, starting with her family doctor and moving through a succession of psychologists and psychiatrists, all to no avail. The problem was that her husband always put on such a good show that *her* account of things was seldom believed. None of these clinicians could see beyond the husband's charming and convincing display. The poor woman began to believe that *she* was the real problem.

Even after a solid diagnosis has been made, your troubles are far from over. The next steps will depend on your particular situation and should be planned with the aid of a competent professional experienced in dealing with psychopaths. State psychiatric and psychological associations usually have a list of clinicians they can recommend. You might also try local mental health and university counseling centers.

• *Don't blame yourself.* Whatever the reasons for your involvement with a psychopath, it is important that you not accept blame for his or her attitudes and behavior. Psychopaths play by the same rules—their rules—with everyone. Of course, your own personality and behavior will have something to do with the specific nature of the interactions that occur. For example, a woman who stands up for her rights may be physically abused, whereas a more submissive woman may spend her life wondering about the whereabouts of her philandering husband. A third woman might walk out at the first sign of trouble and never look back. In each case, the basic problem is having a psychopathic husband in the first place.

Similarly, parents of a psychopathic son or daughter continually agonize over their own role in the development of the disorder. It is very difficult to convince these parents that the chances are they did nothing wrong. Again, they may have ameliorated or exacerbated the situation, but there is no evidence that parental behavior *causes* psychopathy.

• *Be aware of who the victim is.* Psychopaths often give the impression that it is *they* who are suffering and that it is the victims who are to blame for their misery. But they are suffering a lot less than you are, and for different reasons. Don't waste your sympathy on them; their problems are not in the same league as yours. Theirs stem primarily from not getting what they want, whereas yours result from a physical, emotional, or financial pounding.

• *Recognize that you are not alone.* Most psychopaths have lots of victims. It is certain that a psychopath who is causing you grief is also causing grief to others. Tracking them down to exchange stories and information could help you deal with the problem, if only to demonstrate that it is not you who are at fault. Everyone is vulnerable to the psychopath, and there is no shame in being victimized. This may be difficult to accept if you have just been conned and are too embarrassed to complain to the police or to testify in court. But you may be surprised by the number of other people in your community who have been taken in.

• *Be careful about power struggles.* Keep in mind that psychopaths have a strong need for psychological and physical control over others. They must be in charge, and they will use charm, intimidation, and violence to ensure their authority. In a power struggle a psychopath will usually focus on winning. This doesn't mean that you shouldn't stand up for your rights, only that it will probably be difficult to do so without risking serious emotional or physical trauma.

In some cases, you may be able to use the psychopath's "win at all costs" philosophy to your advantage. For example, in a local case a woman and her psychopathic ex-husband were engaged in a prolonged and bitter custody dispute over their two children. The lawyer for the woman, realizing that the man was dangerous, was intent on winning, and didn't actually care about the welfare of the children, advised his client to agree to a joint custody arrangement. This is what the ex-husband had wanted all along, and having "won the battle," he lost all interest in the children. Although the lawyer's tactics worked in this case, he ran a great risk of having the man decide to exercise his right of joint custody, with potentially disastrous consequences for the children.

• *Set firm ground rules.* Although power struggles with a psychopath are risky at best, you may be able to set up some clear ground rules—both for yourself and for the psychopath—to make your life easier and begin the difficult transition from victim to a person looking out for yourself. For example, this may mean that you will no longer bail him or her out of trouble, no matter what the circumstances.

A woman I know was caught in a web of financial manipulation and deceit woven by a glib "consultant." Every time she confronted him, he convinced her that he was working on the problem and that she would soon get back the money he supposedly had invested for her. Finally, in desperation, she decided not to discuss anything with him unless there was a third party present or everything was in writing. It soon became clear to her that she was getting nowhere with him, and she began legal proceedings to recover her money.

Reasonable but firm ground rules—"what you have to do to live here"—may be the only way to preserve your sanity when dealing with a psychopathic son or daughter. These rules must be clear and consistently enforced if they are to stand any chance of having an impact. Specific parenting skills and strategies are outside the scope of this book, but the books listed in the Notes for chapter 12 provide helpful information.

• *Don't expect dramatic changes.* To a large extent, the personalities of psychopaths are "carved in stone." There is little likelihood that anything you do will produce fundamental, sustained changes in how they see themselves or others. They may promise to change and may even show short-term improvements in their behavior, but in most cases you will face years of disappointment if you believe that permanent changes for the better have occurred. Although some psychopaths do "mellow" a bit with age, and as a consequence become somewhat easier to live with, in most cases they remain what they have always been.

The problem is particularly tragic when it is a son or daughter who is psychopathic. In a frantic search for help and understanding, the parents typically find themselves shunted from one professional or agency to another, seldom with satisfactory results. The bewildered parents use an enormous amount of energy and resources in generally unsuccessful attempts to understand and control their child. In most cases, they face years of frustration and demands to bail their son or daughter out of trouble.

• *Cut your losses.* The psychopath may succeed in shattering your self-confidence and may convince you—and your friends— that you are unworthy of his or her time or even that you are "losing it." The more you give in, the more you will be taken advantage of by the psychopath's insatiable appetite for power and control.

Rather than make fruitless attempts to adapt to a hopeless situation—usually by giving in, accepting your lot in life, or losing your self-identity—it may be better to recognize that your emotional and physical survival requires that you take charge of your life. This can be a tricky move—even a dangerous one— and it requires good professional advice, both clinical and legal.

Of course, if you are the parent of a young psychopath, you cannot simply give up on your child. You will have to work closely with teachers, counselors, and clinicians experienced in dealing with psychopathic children, no matter how modest the expected results.

• *Use support groups.* By the time your suspicions have led you to seek a diagnosis, you already know that you're in for a very long and bumpy ride. Make sure you have all the emotional support you can muster.

Many organizations and groups are devoted to helping victims of crime to understand and cope with their plight. In most cases the victim learns that he or she is not alone and is able to share experiences with other victims. For example, most urban areas have crisis centers and support groups concerned with domestic violence, emotionally and behaviorally disturbed children, and victims' rights. Depending on the nature of the problem, one or more of these established groups may be of real benefit to you. But what we really need are support groups specifically designed for the victims of psychopaths. Perhaps this book will help to encourage the development of such groups.

Epilogue

After they have reviewed the literature on a topic it is customary for scientists to conclude with the statement that more research is needed. I will do so, for two reasons.

First, in spite of more than a century of clinical study and speculation and several decades of scientific research, the mystery of the psychopath still remains. Some recent developments have provided us with new insights into the nature of this disturbing disorder, and its borders are becoming more defined. But the fact is, compared with other major clinical disorders, little systematic research has been devoted to psychopathy, even though it is responsible for far more social distress and disruption than all other psychiatric disorders combined.

Second, rather than try to pick up the pieces after the damage has been done, it would make far greater sense to increase our efforts to understand this perplexing disorder and to search for effective early interventions. The alternatives are to continue devoting massive resources to the prosecution, incarceration, and supervision of psychopaths after they have committed offenses against society, and to continue to ignore the welfare and plight of their victims. The criminal justice system spends billions of dollars every year in a vain attempt to "rehabilitate" or "resocialize" psychopaths and other persistent offenders. But these terms—popular with politicians and prison administrators—are little more than buzzwords. We have to learn how to socialize them, not resocialize them. And this will require serious efforts at research and early intervention.

The social and financial costs to society of failing to solve the deadly mystery of the psychopath will be staggering. It is imperative that we continue the search for clues.

Chapter Notes

Introduction

1. Tim Cahill (1987). *Buried Dreams*. New York: Bantam Books.
2. Richard Neville and Julie Clarke (1979). *The Life and Crimes of Charles Sobhraj*. London: Jonathan Cape.
3. Joe McGinniss (1989). *Fatal Vision*. New York: New American Library.
4. James Clarke (1990). *Last Rampage*. New York: Berkley.
5. Darcy O'Brien (1985). *Two of a Kind: The Hillside Stranglers*. New York: New American Library.
6. Clifford Linedecker (1991). *Night Stalker*. New York: St. Martin's Press.
7. Ann Rule (1987). *Small Sacrifices*. New York: New American Library.
8. ———(1980). *The Stranger Beside Me*. New York: Signet.
9. Ian Mulgrew (1990). *Final Payoff*. Toronto, Ontario: Seal Books.
10. Sue Horton (1989). *The Billionaire Boys Club*. New York: St. Martin's Press.
11. Joseph Wambaugh (1987). *Echoes in the Darkness*. New York: Bantam Books.
12. Harry MacLean (1988). *In Broad Daylight*. New York: Dell.
13. Joseph Wambaugh (1989). *The Blooding*. New York: Bantam.
14. Peter Maas (1990). *In a Child's Name*. New York: Pocket Books. Television movie, CBS, November 17, 1991.
15. Gary Provost (1991). *Perfect Husband*. New York: Pocket Books.
16. Dirk Johnson (February 17, 1992). "Jury weary after gruesome testimony." N.Y. Times News Service.
17. Robert Gollmar (1981). *Edward Gein*. New York: Pinnacle Books.

18. Margeret Cheney (1976). *The Co-ed Killer*. New York: Walker & Company.

19. Lawrence Klausner (1981). *Son of Sam*. New York: McGraw-Hill.

Chapter 2. *Focusing the Picture*

1. Robert H. Gollmar (1981). *Edward Gein*. New York: Windsor Publishing Corp. The author was the judge in Gein's trial.

2. American Psychiatric Association (1987). *Diagnostic and Statistical Manual: Mental Disorders* (rev. 3d ed.). Washington, D.C.: Author. The fourth edition (DSM-IV) was published in 1994.

3. The problem was not resolved with the publication of the fourth edition of the DSM in 1994. The American Psychiatric Association conducted field trials to reevaluate the diagnostic criteria for antisocial personality disorder. An essential part of the field trial was the use of a ten-item version of the *Psychopathy Checklist*, described in the next two chapters. Although the field trial confirmed that personality traits could be rated reliably, the diagnostic criteria for antisocial personality disorder in DSM-IV are much as they were in DSM-III-R. The DSM-IV field trial is described by R.D. Hare, S.D. Hart, and T.J. Harpur (1991). *Journal of Abnormal Psychology* 100, 391–98. More detailed accounts and critiques of the field trial can be found in W.J. Livesley (ed.) (1995). *The DSM-IV Personality Disorders*. New York: Guilford.

4. The historical development of the concept of psychopathy has been described in detail by many authors. I have found the following particularly useful: Hervey Cleckley (1976; 5th ed.). *The Mask of Sanity*. St. Louis, MO: Mosby; William McCord and Joan McCord (1964). *The Psychopath: An Essay on the Criminal Mind*. Princeton, NJ: Van Nostrand; Theodore Millon (1981). *Disorders of Personality*. New York: Wiley.

5. Unless otherwise indicated, references to Cleckley's work are from the most recent edition his book: Hervey Cleckley (1976; 5th ed.). *The Mask of Sanity*. St. Louis, MO: Mosby. The book is no longer available from Mosby but can be obtained from

Emily S. Cleckley, Publishers, 3024 Fox Spring Road, Augusta, GA 30903.

6. Drafts of the *Psychopathy Checklist* first were made available to researchers in 1980 and 1985. The most recent version was published in 1991 (see note 1 for chapter 3).

Chapter 3. *The Profile: Feelings and Relationships*

1. The *Psychopathy Checklist* is published by Multi-Health Systems (908 Niagara Falls Blvd, North Tonawanda, NY 14120–2060; in Canada, 65 Overlea Blvd, Toronto, Ontario M4H 1P1) and is available to qualified users. The items in the Psychopathy Checklist are scored by combining interview, case-history, and archival data. However, some investigators have obtained valid scores solely from extensive, good quality file and archival information (e.g., G.T. Harris, M.E. Rice, & C.A. Cormier. Psychopathy and violent recidivism. *Law and Human Behavior*, 1991, 15, 625–637).

2. Joseph Wambaugh (1987). *Echoes in the Darkness.* New York: Bantam Books.

3. Joe McGinniss (1989). *Fatal Vision.* New York: Signet.

4. Ann Rule (1988). *Small Sacrifices.* New York: New American Library. p. 468.

5. Stephen G. Michaud and Hugh Aynesworth (1989). *Ted Bundy: Conversations with a Killer.* New York: New American Library.

6. "The Mind of a Murderer." *Frontline.* PBS, March 27, 1984. Also see D. O'Brien (1985). *Two of a Kind: The Hillside Stranglers.* New York: New American Library; and J. Reid Meloy (1988). *The Psychopathic Mind: Origins, Dynamics, and Treatments.* Northvale, NJ: Jason Aronson, Inc.

7. Quotes are from Tim Cahill (1987). *Buried Dreams.* New York: Bantam.

8. Peter Maas (1990). *In a Child's Name.* New York: Pocket Books.

9. Robert Rieber (1997). *Manufacturing Social Distress: The Psychopathy of Everyday Life.* New York: Plenum.

10. Paul Ekman (1985). *Telling Lies.* New York: Norton.

11. Michaud and Aynesworth (1989). p. 3.
12. From the television program *A Current Affair*, October 10, 1991.
13. From the television program *The Oprah Winfrey Show*, September 26, 1988.
14. J. H. Johns and H.C. Quay (1962). The effect of social reward on verbal conditioning in psychopathic and neurotic military offenders. *Journal of Consulting Psychology* 36, 217–20.
15. Jack Abbott (1981). *In the Belly of the Beast: Letters from Prison.* New York: Random House. p. 13.
16. One of the earliest studies was conducted by David Lykken (1957). A study of anxiety in the sociopathic personality. *Journal of Abnormal Psychology and Social Psychology* 55, 6–10. For a review of the research literature see R. D. Hare (1978). Electrodermal and cardiovascular correlates of psychopathy. In R. D. Hare and D. Schalling (eds.). *Psychopathic Behavior: Approaches to Research.* Chichester, England: Wiley. The most recent study was by J. Ogloff and S. Wong (1990). Electrodermal and cardiovascular evidence of a coping response in psychopaths. *Criminal Justice and Behavior* 17, 231–45. In most of these studies palmar sweating and heart rate were recorded while the subject awaited delivery of a painful electric shock or a loud noise.

Chapter 4. The Profile: Lifestyle

1. William McCord and Joan McCord (1964). *The Psychopath: An Essay on the Criminal Mind.* Princeton, NJ: Van Nostrand. p. 51.
2. *Playboy*, May 1977. p. 80.
3. McCord and McCord (1964). p.9.
4. *Diabolical Minds*. NBC, November 3, 1991. The television program was an *Unsolved Mysteries* special.
5. Ann Rule (1988). *Small Sacrifices*. New York: New American Library.
6. Daniel Goleman. *The New York Times*, August 7, 1991.
7. For example, see D. Olweus, J. Block, and M. Radke-Yarrow (eds) (1986). *Development of Antisocial and Prosocial Behavior*. New York: Academic Press.

8. *Diabolical Minds*. NBC, November 3, 1991.
9. Daniel Goleman. *The New York Times*. July 7, 1987.

Chapter 5. *Internal Controls: The Missing Piece*

1. Robert Hare (1970). *Psychopathy: Theory and Research*. New York: Wiley; Gordon Trasler (1978). Relations between psychopathy and persistent criminality. In R.D. Hare & D. Schalling (eds.). *Psychopathic Behavior: Approaches to Research*. Chichester, England: Wiley.
2. A. R. Luria (1973). *The Working Brain*. New York: Basic Books.
3. Ethan Gorenstein (1991). A cognitive perspective on antisocial personality. In P. Magaro (ed.). *Annual Review of Psychopathology: Cognitive Bases of Mental Disorders*, vol. 1. Newbury Park, CA: Sage.
4. Joanne Intrator. Personal communication, October 1991.
5. Robert Lindner (1944). *Rebel Without a Cause*. New York: Grune and Stratton. The book went on to become an affecting 1955 movie of the same name, but Lindner's ideas about psychopathy never made it to the screen.
6. Jose Sanchez. Quoted in *The New York Times*, July 7, 1989.

Chapter 6. *Crime: The Logical Choice*

1. Discussions of the causes of crime are presented by James Wilson and Richard Herrenstein (1985). *Crime and Human Nature*. New York: Touchstone.
2. An analysis of the attractions that crime has for some individuals is given by Jack Kratz (1988). *Seductions of Crime*. New York: Basic Books.
3. R. D. Hare, K. Strachan, and A. E. Forth (1993). Psychopathy and crime: A review. In K. Howells and C. Hollin (eds.). *Clinical Approaches to Mentally Disordered Offenders*. New York: Wiley.
4. Tim Cahill (1987). *Buried Dreams*. New York: Bantam Books.

5. Normal Mailer (1980). *The Executioner's Song*. New York: Warner Books.

6. *Playboy,* May 1977. p. 76.

7. R. D. Hare and L. N. McPherson (1984). Violent and aggressive behavior by criminal psychopaths. *International Journal of Law and Psychiatry* 7, 35–50; D. S. Kosson, S. S. Smith, and J. P. Newman (1990). Evaluating the construct validity of psychopathy on Black and White male inmates: Three preliminary studies. *Journal of Abnormal Psychology* 99, 250–59; R. C. Serin (1991). Psychopathy and violence in criminals. *Journal of Interpersonal Violence* 6, 423–31; S. Wong (1984). Criminal and institutional behaviors of psychopaths. *Programs Branch Users Report.* Ottawa, Ontario, Canada: Ministry of the Solicitor-General of Canada.

8. *Playboy,* May 1977. p. 76.

9. S. Williamson, R. Hare, and S. Wong (1987). Violence: Criminal psychopaths and their victims. *Canadian Journal of Behavioral Science* 1, 454–62.

10. Quoted by Felicia Lee. *N.Y. Times News Service,* November 26, 1991.

11. R. Prentky and R. Knight (1991). Identifying critical dimensions for discriminating among rapists. *Journal of Consulting and Clinical Psychology,* 59, 643–661.

12. Rapist "might murder." *The Province,* Vancouver, B.C., January 28, 1987.

13. T. Newlove, S. Hart, and D. Dutton (1992). *Psychopathy and Family Violence.* Unpublished manuscript. Department of Psychology, University of British Columbia, Vancouver, Canada.

14. C. P. Ewing (1983). "Dr. death" and the case for an ethical ban on psychiatric and psychological predictions of dangerousness in capital sentencing proceedings. *American Journal of Law and Medicine* 8, 407–28.

15. S. D. Hart, P. R. Kropp, and R. D. Hare (1988). Performance of male psychopaths following conditional release from prison. *Journal of Consulting and Clinical Psychology* 56, 227–32; R. C. Serin, R. D. Peters, and H. E. Barbaree (1990). Predictors of psychopathy and release outcome in a criminal population. *Psy-*

chological Assessment: A Journal of Consulting and Clinical Psychology 2, 419–22.

16. M. E. Rice, G. T. Harris, and V. L. Quinsey (1990). A follow-up of rapists assessed in a maximum security psychiatric facility. *Journal of Interpersonal Violence* 4, 435–48.

17. The first to do so was Atascadero State Hospital, Atascadero, California. (David Plate, Chief of Psychology, personal communication, November 27, 1991.)

18. J. E. Donovan, R. Jessor, and F. M. Costa (1988). Syndrome of problem behavior in adolescence: A replication. *Journal of Consulting and Clinical Psychology* 56, 762–65; R. Loeber (1988). Natural histories of conduct problems, delinquency, and associated substance abuse: Evidence for developmental progressions. In B. Lahey and A. E. Kazdin (eds.). *Advances in Clinical Child Psychology*, vol. 11. New York: Plenum; D. Olweus, J. Block, and M. Radke-Yarrow (eds.) (1986). *Development of Antisocial and Prosocial Behavior*. New York: Academic Press.

19. R. D. Hare, L. N. McPherson, and A. E. Forth (1988). Male psychopaths and their criminal careers. *Journal of Consulting and Clinical Psychology* 56, 710–14; G. T. Harris, M. E. Rice, and C. A. Cormier (1991). Psychopathy and violent recidivism. *Law and Human Behavior* 15, 625–37; L. N. Robins (1966). *Deviant Children Grown Up*, Baltimore, MD: Williams & Wilkins.

Chapter 7. *White-Collar Psychopaths*

1. Daniel Goleman. *The New York Times*, July 7, 1987.

2. Letter from Brian Rosner, Office of the District Attorney of the County of New York, July 15, 1987. Rosner is now with the firm of King and Spalding, New York.

3. Ed Cony. *Wall Street Journal*, March 23, 1987. p. 1.

4. The People of the State of New York Against John A. Grambling, Indictment No. 2800/85. *Proceedings.* Supreme Court of the State of New York, County of New York Criminal Term, Part 48; The People of the State of New York Against John A. Grambling, Indictment No. 2800/85. *Sentencing Memorandum;* Letter from John A. Grambling to the Honorable Herman Cahn, New York Supreme Court, March 6, 1987.

5. Brian Rosner (1990). *Swindle.* Homewood, IL: Business One Irwin.

6. The People of the State of New York Against John A. Grambling, Indictment No. 2800/85. *Sentencing Memorandum.*

7. *Sentencing Memorandum.* p. 69.

8. *Sentencing Memorandum.* p. 78.

9. *Sentencing Memorandum.* p. 81 (emphasis is in the letter written by the father-in-law).

10. *Sentencing Memorandum.* p.3.

11. John Grambling, Jr. Letter to Justice Cahn, March 6, 1987. p. 30.

12. *Proceedings.* p. 54.

13. *Proceedings.* p. 51.

14. *Sentencing Memorandum.* p. 10.

15. *Sentencing Memorandum.* p. 11.

16. Brian Rosner (1990).

17. *Sentencing Memorandum.* p. 38.

18. B. Bearak. *Los Angeles Times,* March 10, 1986. pp. 1, 12.

19. Max Lerner. "How grateful should Europe be?" *Actions and Passions* (1949). Quotation no. 199.7 in R. Thomas Tripp (1970). *The International Thesaurus of Quotations.* New York: Harper & Row.

20. Jonathan Beaty and S. C. Gwynne. "The Dirtiest Bank of All." *Time,* July 29, 1991. p. 28.

21. John Grambling, Jr. Letter to the Honorable Herman Cahn, New York Supreme Court, County of New York: Part 48. March 6, 1987. The letter was an attempt to convince Justice Cahn that he, Grambling, did not warrant a long sentence for his crimes.

22. Justice Herman Cahn. *Proceedings.* p. 55.

23. Brian Rosner. *Sentencing Memorandum.* pp. 84–85.

Chapter 8. *Words from an Overcoat Pocket*

1. *Inside Edition.* November 22, 1990.

2. Stephen G. Michaud and Hugh Aynesworth (1989). *Ted Bundy:*

Conversations with a Killer. New York: New American Library. p. 107.

3. From an article by Peter Worthington, *Saturday Night,* July–August, 1993.

4. N. Geschwind and A. Galaburda (1987). *Cerebral Lateralization: Biological Mechanisms, Associations, and Pathology.* Cambridge, MA: MIT Press.

5. R. D. Hare and L. N. McPherson (1984). Psychopathy and perceptual asymmetry during verbal dichotic listening. *Journal of Abnormal Psychology* 93, 141–49.; R. D. Hare and J. Jutai (1988). Psychopathy and cerebral asymmetry in semantic processing. *Personality and Individual Differences* 9, 329–37.; A. Raine, M. O'Brien, N. Smiley, A. Scerbo, and C. Chan (1990). Reduced lateralization in verbal dichotic listening in adolescent psychopaths. *Journal of Abnormal Psychology* 99, 272–77.

6. J. H. Johns and H. C. Quay (1962). The effect of social reward on verbal conditioning in psychopaths and neurotic military offenders. *Journal of Consulting Psychology* 26, 217–20.

7. V. Grant (1977). *The Menacing Stranger.* New York: Dabor Science Publications. p. 50.

8. W. Johnson (1946). *People in Quandaries: The Semantics of Personal Adjustment.* New York: Harper & Brothers.

9. Hervey Cleckley (1976; 5th ed.). *The Mask of Sanity.* St. Louis, MO: Mosby, p. 230.

10. S. Williamson, T. J. Harpur, and R. D. Hare (1991). Abnormal processing of affective words by psychopaths. *Psychophysiology* 28, 260–73. This is the "brain wave" study referred to in the Introduction.

11. ———— (August 1990). *Sensitivity to emotional polarity in psychopaths.* Paper presented at meeting of the American Psychological Association, Boston, MA.

12. Diane Downs (1989). *Best Kept Secrets.* Springfield, OR: Danmark Publishing.

13. R. Day and S. Wong (1993). *Psychopaths process emotion in the left hemisphere.* Manuscript submitted for publication.

14. Michaud and Aynesworth (1989). p. 158.

15. Discussions of language-related hand gestures are provided by P. Feyereisen (1983). Manual activity during speaking in apha-

sic subjects. *International Journal of Psychology* 18, 545–56; D. McNeill (1985). So you think gestures are nonverbal. *Psychology Review* 91, 332–50; B. Rime and L. Schiaratura (1988). Gesture and speech. In R. Feldman and B. Rime (eds.). *Fundamentals of Nonverbal Behavior.* New York: Cambridge University Press.

16. B. Gillstrom and R. D. Hare (1988). Language-related hand gestures in psychopaths. *Journal of Personality Disorders,* 2, 21–27; also see B. Rime, H. Bouvy, B. Leborgne, and F. Rouillon (1978). Psychopathy and nonverbal behavior in an interpersonal situation. *Journal of Abnormal Psychology* 87, 636–43.

17. Paul Ekman (1985). *Telling Lies.* New York: Norton.

18. Julius Charles Hare and Augustus William Hare (1827). *Guesses at Truth.* Quotation No. 329.21 in R. Thomas Tripp (1970). *The International Thesaurus of Quotations.* New York: Harper & Row.

19. Sherrie Williamson (1991). *Cohesion and Coherence in the Speech of Psychopaths.* Unpublished doctoral dissertation. University of British Columbia, Vancouver, Canada.

20. Material and quotes are from Terry Ganey (1989). *St. Joseph's Children: A True Story of Terror and Justice.* New York: Carol Publishing Group.

21. Material and quotes are from Tim Cahill (1987). *Buried Dreams.* New York: Bantam Books.

Chapter 9. *Flies in the Web*

1. B. Rime and L. Schiaratura (1990). Gesture and speech. In R. Feldman and B. Rime (eds.). *Fundamentals of Nonverbal Behavior.* New York: Cambridge University Press.

2. Joseph Wambaugh (1987). *Echoes in the Darkness.* New York: Bantam Books. pp. 22–23.

3. Clifford Linedecker (1991). *Night Stalker.* New York: St. Martin's Press. pp. 202–203.

4. Robert Mason Lee. "Bambi: The face of a killer." *The Sun,* Vancouver, Canada, November 3, 1990; Kris Radish (1992). *Run, Bambi, Run: The Beautiful Ex-Cop Convicted of Murder Who Escaped to Freedom and Won America's Heart.* New York: Carol Publishing

Group. Lawrencia Bambenek (1992). *Woman on Trial.* Toronto: Harper Collins.

5. Personal communication, April 1991.

6. Some case histories of women attracted to convicted killers are presented by Sheila Isenberg (1991). *Women Who Love Men Who Kill.* New York: Simon & Schuster. The psychological forces at play in those who form associations with violent individuals are discussed by J. Reid Meloy (1992). *Violent Attachments.* Northvale, NJ: Jason Aronson, Inc.

Chapter 10. *The Roots of the Problem*

1. Stories of adopted children who wreak havoc on their new families are not uncommon. However, most accounts of the early manifestations of psychopathy are provided by the biological parents of the children involved.

2. Longitudinal studies of the progression of psychopathy and antisocial behavior from childhood to adulthood include: Lee N. Robins (1966). *Deviant Children Grow Up.* Baltimore, MA: Williams & Wilkins; David Farrington (1991). Antisocial personality from childhood to adulthood. *The Psychologist* 4, 389–94.

3. A review of the research literature on this topic was provided by B. Lahey, K. McBurnett, R. Loeber, and E. Hart (1995). Psychobiology of Conduct Disorder. In G. P. Sholevar (ed.). *Conduct Disorders in Children and Adolescents: Assessments and Interventions.* Washington, D.C.: American Psychiatric Press.

4. This research is described in detail by P.J. Frick, B.S. O'Brien, J.A. Wooton, and K. McBurnett (1994). Psychopathy and conduct problems in children. *Journal of Abnormal Psychology* 103, 700–07.

5. Rolf Loeber (1990). Development and Risk Factors of Juvenile Antisocial Behavior and Delinquency. *Clinical Psychology Review* 10, 1–41; David Farrington (1991). Antisocial personality from childhood to adulthood. *The Psychologist* 4, 389–94.

6. Ken Magid and Carole A. McKelvey (1989). *High Risk: Children Without Conscience.* New York: Bantam.

7. "Officials stymied by alleged rapist, 9." *Seattle Times,* July 21, 1992.

8. See J. MacMillan and L. K. Kofoed (1984). Sociobiology and antisocial behavior. *Journal of Mental and Nervous Diseases* 172, 701–06; H. C. Harpending and J. Sobus (1987). Sociopathy as an adaptation. *Ethology and Sociobiology* 8, 63S–72S.

9. Ann Rule (1987). *Small Sacrifices*. New York: New American Library. Also revealing is the book written by Diane Downs (1989). *Best Kept Secrets*. Springfield, OR: Danmark Publishing.

10. See R. D. Hare (1970). *Psychopathy: Theory and Research*. New York: Wiley.

11. Robert Kegan (1986). The child behind the mask: Sociopathy as developmental delay. In W. H. Reid, D. Dorr, J. I. Walker, and J. W. Bonner, III. *Unmasking the Psychopath*. New York: W. W. Norton.

12. R. D. Hare (1984). Performance of psychopaths on cognitive tasks related to frontal lobe function. *Journal of Abnormal Psychology* 93, 133–40; S. D. Hart, A. E. Forth, and R. D. Hare (1990). Performance of male psychopaths on selected neuropsychological tests. *Journal of Abnormal Psychology* 99, 374–79; J. J. Hoffman, R. W. Hall, and T. W. Bartsch (1987). On the relative importance of "Psychopathic" personality and alcoholism on neuropsychological measures of frontal lobe dysfunction. *Journal of Abnormal Psychology* 96, 158–60.

13. See E. E. Gorenstein and J. P. Newman (1980). Disinhibitory psychopathology: A new perspective and model for research. *Psychological Review* 87, 301–315; J. P. Newman (1987). Reaction to punishment in extroverts and psychopaths: Implications for the impulsive behavior of disinhibited individuals. *Journal of Research in Personality* 21, 464–80; A. R. Damasio, D. Tranel, and H. Damasio (1990). Individuals with sociopathic behavior caused by frontal damage fail to respond autonomically to social stimuli. *Behavioral Brain Research* 41, 81–94.

Damage to the front parts of the brain can produce several psychopathic-like behaviors, including poor judgment and planning ability, impulsivity, failure to be influenced by punishment, and poor social conduct. However, this "acquired psychopathy," as some investigators refer to the condition, is quite different from the distinct set of personality traits and behaviors that defines psychopathy. Nevertheless, the study of brain-damaged patients may provide clues to the nature of psychopathy.

14. Reviews of early risk factors for adult problems, including criminality and violence, have been provided by several investigators. See, for example, C. S. Widom (1989). The Cycle of Violence. *Science* 244, 160–66; D. Olweus, J. Block, and M. Radke-Yarrow (eds.) (1986). *Development of Antisocial and Prosocial Behavior*. New York: Academic Press; R. Loeber (1990). Development and Risk Factors of Juvenile Antisocial Behavior and Delinquency. *Clinical Psychology Review* 10, 1–41; J. McCord (1988). Parental behavior in the cycle of aggression. *Psychiatry* 51, 14–23; Adrian Raine (1988). Antisocial Behavior and Social Psychophysiology. In H. L. Wagner (ed.). *Social Psychophysiology and Emotion: Theory and Clinical Applications*. New York: Wiley.

15. Magid now views psychopathy as the result of both biological and social factors. *Personal Communication*, July 22, 1993.

16. In their influential 1964 book, *The Psychopath: An Essay on the Criminal Mind*. (Princeton, NJ: Van Nostrand), William and Joan McCord argued that social factors were a major cause of psychopathy. Recently, Joan McCord had this to say about the problem: "Both parental rejection and inconsistent punitiveness have been implicated in the etiology of psychopathy. . . . (But) the data have been retrospective and the behavior of the psychopath might well have caused, rather than resulted from, parental rejection" (July 1984). *Family Sources of Crime*. Paper presented at the meeting of the International Society for Research on Aggression. Turku, Finland; also see J. McCord (1988). Parental behavior in the cycle of aggression. *Psychiatry* 51, 14–23.

17. Some recent discussions of the evidence that individual differences in intelligence, aptitudes, and personality are associated with genetic variation include the following: T. J. Bouchard, D. T. Lykken, M. McGue, N. L. Segal, and A. Tellegen (1990). Sources of human psychological differences: The Minnesota study of twins reared apart. *Science* 250, 223–28; T. J. Bouchard and M. McGue (1990). Genetic and rearing environmental influences on adult personality: An analysis of adopted twins reared apart. Special Issue: Biological foundations of personal-

ity: Evolution, behavioral genetics, and psychophysiology. *Journal of Personality* 58, 263–92; J. E. Bates and M. K. Rothbart (eds.) (1989). *Temperament in Childhood*. New York: Wiley; J. Kagan, J. S. Resnick, and N. Snidman (1988). Biological bases of childhood shyness. *Science* 240, 167–71; J. Kagan and N. Snidman (1991). Infant predictors of inhibited and uninhibited profiles. *Psychological Science* 2, 40–44. A discussion relating anxiety to adolescent psychopathy is given by B. Lahey, K. McBurnett, R. Loeber, and E. Hart (1995). Psychobiology of Conduct Disorder. In G. P. Sholevar (ed.). *Conduct Disorders in Children and Adolescents: Assessments and Interventions*. Washington, D.C.: American Psychiatric Press.

18. Evidence from family, twin, and adoption studies indicates that criminality and violence in general, and psychopathy in particular, are at least influenced by genetic and biological contributions to temperament, and shaped by environmental and social forces. For example, see S. A. Mednick, T. E. Moffitt, and S. A. Stack (eds.) (1987). *The Causes of Crime: New Biological Approaches*. Cambridge, England: Cambridge University Press; R. Plomin, J. C. DeFries, and D. W. Fulker (1988). *Nature and Nurture During Infancy and Early Childhood*. Cambridge, England: Cambridge University Press; F. Schulsinger (1974). Psychopathy, heredity, and environment. In S. A. Mednick, F. Schulsinger, J. Higgins, and B. Bell (eds.). *Genetics, Environment, and Psychopathology* [pp. 177–95]. Amsterdam: North Holland/Elsevier. Of particular importance is a recent twin study that found evidence for a strong genetic contribution to the cluster of personality traits (described in chapter 3) that define psychopathy (W. J. Livesley, K. L. Jang, D. N. Jackson, and P. A. Vernon. *Genetic and Environmental Contributions to Dimensions of Personality Disorder*. Paper presented at Meeting of the American Psychiatric Association, Washington, D.C., May 2–7, 1992; Adrian Raine (1988). Antisocial Behavior and Social Psychophysiology. In H. L. Wagner (ed.). *Social Psychophysiology and Emotion: Theory and Clinical Applications*. New York: Wiley.

19. E. DeVita, A. E. Forth, and R. D. Hare (June 1990). *Psychopathy, family background, and early criminality*. Paper presented at meeting of the Canadian Psychological Association, Ottawa, Canada.

20. The case was reported by Mary Lynn Young in *The Sun*, Van-

couver, British Columbia, December 12, 1990. The quotations are from this article.

Chapter 11. *The Ethics of Labeling*

1. Atascadero State Hospital in Atascadero, California. Details provided by David Plate, head of psychology (personal communication, August 1991).
2. Ron Rosenbaum (May 1990). Travels with Dr. Death. *Vanity Fair.*
3. Charles P. Ewing (1983). "Dr. Death" and the case for an ethical ban on psychiatric and psychological predictions of dangerousness in capital sentencing proceedings. *American Journal of Law & Medicine* 8, 407–28.

Chapter 12. *Can Anything Be Done?*

1. Robert Hare (1970). *Psychopathy: Theory and Research.* New York: Wiley. p. 110.
2. J. S. Maxmen (1986). *Essential Psychopathology.* New York: W. W. Norton.
3. The treatment program is described by J. R. Ogloff, S. Wong, and A. Greenwood (1990). Treating criminal psychopaths in a therapeutic community program. *Behavioral Sciences and the Law* 8, 81–90. Recidivism following release from the program was determined by J. Hemphill (1991). *Recidivism of Criminal Psychopaths After Therapeutic Community Treatment.* Unpublished masters thesis, Department of Psychology, University of Saskatchewan, Saskatoon, Canada.
4. G. T. Harris, M. E. Rice, and C. A. Cormier (1991). Psychopathy and violent recidivism. *Law and Human Behavior* 15, 625–37.
5. William McCord (1982). *The Psychopath and Millieu Therapy.* New York: Academic Press. p. 202.
6. There are many books that describe procedures and programs for dealing with behavioral problems in children. A few are listed below:
   • E. A. Blechman (1985). *Solving Child Behavior Problems at Home*

and at School. Champaign, IL: Research Press. A workbook approach to common behavioral problems.

- S. W. Garber, M. D. Garber, and R. F. Spitzman (1987). *Good Behavior: Over 1200 Sensible Solutions to Your Child's Problems from Birth to Age Twelve.* New York: Villard Books. An excellent reference for many common child behavioral problems. Covers basic behavioral principles and preventive strategies. Also includes sections on more serious behavioral problems and disorders and gives advice on how to seek professional help.
- H. Kohl (1981). *Growing with Your Children.* New York: Bantam. A practical guide for parents. Deals with such issues as discipline, violence, self-image, and fairness.
- J. Wyckoff and B. C. Unell (1984). *Discipline Without Shouting or Spanking: Practical Solutions to the Most Common Preschool Behavior Problems.* New York: Meadowbrook Books. A practical book that describes common misbehaviors of preschoolers (e.g., temper tantrums, sibling rivalry, messiness, resisting bedtime).
- E. A. Kirby and L. K. Grimley (1986). *Understanding and Treating Attention Deficit Disorder.* New York: Pergamon Press. A good resource book for parents trying to deal with a hyperactive child.

7. Robert Hare (1992). *A Model Treatment Program for Offenders at High Risk for Violence.* Ottawa, Canada: Research Branch, Correctional Service of Canada.

Chapter 13. *A Survival Guide*

1. For a discussion of the psychopath's "predatory stare" see J. Reid Meloy (1988). *The Psychopathic Mind.* Northvale, NJ: Aronson, Inc.

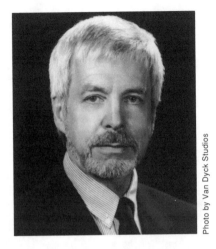

Robert D. Hare, Ph.D., considered one of the world's foremost experts in the area of psychopathy, is a professor of psychology at the University of British Columbia. There he developed the Psychopathy Checklist, which is rapidly being adopted worldwide as the standard instrument for researchers and clinicians. Dr. Hare has written two previous books, and numerous articles, on psychopathy.